Contents

Acknowledgements 2

Contributors 3

Preface 5

Foreword 6

Chapter 1: Intellectual disabilities and mental health 7
Raghu Raghavan

Chapter 2: Anxiety disorders in people with intellectual disabilities 21
Tonye Sikabofori and Anupama Iyer

Chapter 3: Depressive disorders in people with intellectual disabilities. 51
Tonye Sikabofori and Anupama Iyer

Chapter 4: User views and experiences 75
Eddie Chaplin and Steve Hardy

Chapter 5: Case formulation 89
Barry Ingham

Chapter 6: Psychopharmacological approaches 105
Caroline Reid and Shoumitro Deb

Chapter 7: Cognitive therapy 125
Dave Dagnan

Chapter 8: Solution focused brief therapy 141
E Veronica (Vicky) Bliss

Chapter 9: Psychodynamic perspective 159
Nadja Alim

Chapter 10: Supporting families 191
Ereny Gobrial and Raghu Raghavan

Chapter 11: Case management and the care programme approach 207
Eddie Chaplin and Steve Hardy

Chapter 12: Intensive support teams 221
Sue Freeman and Philip Reynolds

Acknowledgements

I am very grateful to all people with intellectual disabilities and their families who have helped me to conceptualise the theme of this book. This title would also not have been possible without the help and support of the contributors on the various therapeutic approaches. I extend my thanks to Jan Alcoe and Kerry Boettcher from Pavilion Publishing for commissioning this publication, and I am very grateful to Michael Benge, also from Pavilion Publishing, for his help with the copyediting of the book.

Anxiety and Depression in People with Intellectual Disabilities

Advances in interventions

Edited by Raghu Raghavan

Pavilion

Professional

Anxiety and Depression in People with Intellectual Disabilities: Advances in interventions

© Raghu Raghavan

Published by:
Pavilion Publishing and Media Ltd
Rayford House
School Road
Hove BN3 5HX
UK
Tel: 01273 434943
Fax: 01273 227308
Email: info@pavpub.com
Web: www.pavpub.com

Published 2012

ISBN: 978-1-908066-63-3

Pavilion is the leading publisher and provider of professional development products in the health, social care, education and community safety sectors. We believe that everyone has the right to fulfil their potential and we strive to supply products and services that help raise standards, promote best practices and support continuing professional development.

Editor: Mike Benge, Pavilion Publishing and Media Ltd
Cover design: Emma Garbutt, Pavilion Publishing and Media Ltd
Page layout and typesetting: Anthony Pitt, Pavilion Publishing and Media Ltd
Printer: CMP (uk) Limited

Contributors

Raghu Raghavan Reader in disability and mental health, School of Health, Community and Education Studies, Northumbria University, Newcastle upon Tyne, NE7 7XA.

Nadja Alim Senior psychologist, Lewisham Community Team for Adults with Learning Disabilities, South London and Maudsley NHS Foundation Trust, London.

E Veronica (Vicky) Bliss Brief Therapy Support Services Ltd, Clarks Cottage, Union Lane, Pilling, Lancashire.

Eddie Chaplin Research and strategy lead, Behavioural and Developmental Psychiatry Clinical Academic Group, Institute of Psychiatry, De Crespigny Park, London.

Dave Dagnan Consultant clinical psychologist/clinical director, Cumbria Partnership NHS Foundation Trust and Lancaster University, Community Learning Disability Services, Unit 1, Lakeland Business Centre, Jubilee Road, Workington.

Shoumitro Deb MBBS, FRCPsych, MD, consultant psychiatrist and clinical professor of neuropsychiatry and intellectual disability, University of Birmingham.

Sue Freeman Nurse consultant in learning disability, Intensive Support Service, Northamptonshire Healthcare Foundation, Berrywood Hospital, Berrywood Drive, Northampton.

Ereny Gobrial Lecturer, School of Education, Zagazig University, Egypt.

Steve Hardy Education and training lead, Department of Forensic and Neurodevelopmental Science (FANS), Institute of Psychiatry, King's College London, De Crespigny Park, London.

Barry Ingham Consultant clinical psychologist, Learning Disability Directorate, Northumberland Tyne and Wear Foundation NHS Trust, Morpeth, Northumberland.

Anupama Iyer Consultant in adolescent developmental disabilities, St Andrew's Healthcare, Billing Road, Northampton.

Caroline Reid MBBS, MRCPsych, specialty registrar in psychiatry of learning disabilities, Coventry and Warwickshire Partnership NHS Trust.

Philip Reynolds Principal clinical psychologist, Intensive Support Service, Northamptonshire Healthcare Foundation, Berrywood Hospital, Berrywood Drive, Northampton.

Tonye Sikabofori Consultant psychiatrist in intellectual disabilities, Intensive Support Service, Northamptonshire Healthcare Foundation, Berrywood Hospital, Berrywood Drive, Northampton.

Preface

'Thousands of candles can be lit from a single candle and the life of the candle will not be shortened. Happiness never decreases by being shared.'
Siddhartha Gautama

This book will focus on intervention strategies for treating anxiety and depression in people with intellectual disabilities (ID). The rationale for this theme is the lack of an adequate evidence base for assessment and intervention approaches for this population. For example, although anxiety disorders are among the most common psychiatric disorders in the general population, very little is known about their incidence and manifestation in people with ID. Furthermore, research evidence indicates a high prevalence of depression and related illnesses in this population, and the nature and manifestation of depressive illnesses in people with ID warrant an in-depth examination to highlight the knowledge base of appropriate assessments and intervention strategies. This book explores the full range of anxiety and depressive illnesses in relation to people with ID, captures their nature and manifestation, and describes assessment and intervention approaches.

Developing evidence-based practice is a key theme of the book, and we have focused on the conceptual models for therapeutic interventions for anxiety and depression. The lack of a significant systematic evidence base for effective interventions for people with ID with anxiety and depression continues to challenge all health and social care professionals working with this client group. As the care of people with ID and mental health needs is more complex, it is useful to reflect on the rich and diverse ways that we work with this group to develop a model of practice-based evidence.

We believe that through the consolidation of the evidence base for interventions and services, professionals will be able to plan and develop therapeutic and person-centred care for people with ID.

Foreword

Mental health problems for people with intellectual disabilities remain a serious problem for service users, families, carers and professionals, and mood disorders such as anxiety and depression are of particular concern as they are increasingly recognised as a significant source of distress and are more common than previously accepted.

Anxiety and depression might be presented as distinct clinical entities, or they may overlap and interrelate (Stavrakaki & Lunsky, 2007), and their diagnosis is further complicated by the cognitive and communication difficulties present in people with intellectual disabilities, particularly for those with more severe difficulties (Hurtley, 2006), which raises the risk of misdiagnosis or that these conditions will go unrecognised. Some studies, for example, have suggested that anxiety and depression might be presented as challenging behaviours, while others have expressed doubt about this suggestion (Hurley, 2006).

However, recent progress in conceptualisation, diagnostic methods and therapeutic interventions has advanced our understanding, knowledge and identification of this area, and the increasing participation of service users, their families and their carers has enriched the range of supports available to them.

This book is an important addition to our knowledge of the field, addressing best practice and training with important contributions from service users. Personal experience of a range of different interventions is presented and blended together with evidence-based practice whenever possible. It is hoped that this book will be an essential tool and will decisively contribute to improving practices and facilitating training in an important area that is of great concern to all those supporting people with intellectual disabilities.

Nick Bouras, MD. PhD, FRCPsych
Professor Emeritus of Psychiatry
Programme Director Maudsley International
King's College London
Institute of Psychiatry
London SE5 8AF

Hurley A (2006) Mood disorders in intellectual disability. *Current Opinion in Psychiatry* **19** (5) 465–469.

Stavrakaki C & Lunsky Y (2007) Depression, anxiety and adjustment disorders in people with intellectual disabilities. In: N Bouras and G Holt (Eds) *Psychiatric and Behavioural Disorders in Intellectual and Developmental Disabilities*. Cambridge: Cambridge University Press.

Chapter 1

Intellectual disabilities and mental health

Raghu Raghavan

Overview

This chapter will examine health and social policy with special reference to people with intellectual disabilities (ID) in the UK, and explore the severe health inequalities they experience. It will also discuss the need for psychological and other therapies for people with ID who have mental health needs.

Learning objectives

- To contextualise health and social care policy directives.
- To highlight health inequalities and discrimination.
- To explore resilience and interventions.

Introduction

Community living has laid to rest the myth that the emotional problems experienced by people with ID are the result of institutionalisation alone, and that living in the community would somehow 'remove' or 'cure' such problems. In fact, living in the community has created additional problems for people with ID, such as negative attitudes, social exclusion and a lack of appropriate and meaningful employment. For many people with ID this has also resulted in increased exposure to alcohol and illicit drugs, and made them more vulnerable to abuse and exploitation. Furthermore, the lack of leisure and social opportunities, and a lack of adequate help and support to allow them to access and fully participate in such activities in the community, frustrates many people with ID. Such stressors, when combined with the limited coping and problem solving skills often found in this population, are likely to result in maladaptive ways of coping and mental health problems. However, it is a sad fact that many mental health disorders, such as anxiety and depression, often go unrecognised due to the phenomenon of diagnostic overshadowing – the assumption that mental disorder and ID are mutually exclusive categories rather than ones that overlap.

In fact, research evidence over the last two decades consistently shows that around 40% of people with ID experience a range of mental health disorders during their lives, and that for most of the common mental health disorders, the estimated prevalence in people with ID is far higher than the general population.

Another issue in diagnosis is that people with ID often show severe behaviour problems or challenging behaviours, which pose a serious challenge to services (Emerson, 2001), but the boundaries between such challenging behaviour and mental health disorders has a significant impact on detection and diagnosis. For example, the violent behaviour sometimes apparent in paranoid schizophrenia, and the social withdrawal accompanying clinical depression, can both be described as challenging behaviour. The problems of differential diagnosis of challenging behaviour and mental health disorder may therefore have serious consequences in understanding the therapeutic needs of people with ID.

The extent of this overlap between challenging behaviour and mental health disorders has been examined from different perspectives and been the subject of many debates. Moss *et al* (2000) conducted a study to determine the proportion of people with challenging behaviour who have additional psychiatric symptoms. They surveyed 320 people with ID, with and without challenging behaviour, for the presence of psychiatric symptoms using the Psychiatric Assessment Schedule for Adults with a Developmental Disability Checklist (PAS-ADD) (Moss *et al*, 1998). Their results indicate that an increasing severity of challenging behaviour is associated with increased prevalence of psychiatric symptoms. For example, the study found that depression is four times as prevalent in people whose challenging behaviour was more demanding than in people showing less challenging behaviour. Based on this association, Moss *et al* (2000) highlight that there may be many people with ID and challenging behaviour who may also have unrecognised psychiatric symptoms.

The complex nature of this overlap should therefore be taken into account when diagnosing mental health disorders in this population. Dosen (1993) argues that the area of overlap is broad and that this should not be a reason to abandon efforts to distinguish between challenging behaviour and mental health disorders. Multidisciplinary assessment processes using both behavioural observation and psychological states may therefore be the best option for establishing appropriate diagnoses and treatments.

Policy directions

The Department of Health's *Valuing People* white paper (DH, 2001) and its recent update *Valuing People Now* (DH, 2009) outline the strategy for improving the lives of people with ID and their families. The agenda is based on the recognition of their rights as citizens to be socially included, and to have choice in their daily lives and opportunities to achieve independence. In many respects, *Valuing People* challenged the way services are organised for people with ID, and more importantly the way in which professionals and other service providers work with this population.

Some of the key changes in this area that we have seen over the past decade include:

- the development of real partnerships between services and people with ID and their families, thus promoting inclusion
- a focus on the health of people with ID and the need to improve their health and well-being through focused action, such as the health improvement plans and health facilitators
- the availability of easy-read information on all aspects of health and social care, enabling and empowering people with ID and their families to make informed choices
- increasing the range of housing options and the closure of the NHS campus service provisions
- promoting a personalisation agenda, underpinned by the principles of person-centred planning, by working in partnership with the user and a range of service providers in the locality
- increasing employment opportunities for people with ID.

These initiatives need to be fully supported and maintained to observe their long-term impact on improving the lives of people with ID.

With regard to mental health needs, *Valuing People* highlighted that most psychiatric disorders are common in people with ID and suggested that the *National Service Framework for Mental Health* (DH, 1999) was applicable to people with ID of working age. *Valuing People* advocated the use of mainstream mental health services in combination with a range of specialist services for people with ID.

The service structures for people with ID who experience mental health disorders are fraught with confusion, complexity and conflict: confusion in terms of the nature and manifestation of mental health problems in people with ID; complexity in terms of the challenges for appropriate detection, diagnosis and intervention approaches; and conflict in terms of the service structures and processes that work against the needs and wishes of users and their carers. As a result, people with ID and mental health needs face severe inequalities. What is required is a truly inclusive mainstream service accepting people with ID and mental health needs and offering appropriate therapeutic services.

However, mainstream mental health services continue to pose major barriers for people with ID, whose experiences of such services are far from satisfactory. One of most common uses of mainstream services by people with ID is the admission to general adult wards in mental health hospitals, where they experience a number of problems:

- Many find the general psychiatric wards too busy, chaotic and threatening, having come from quieter protected environments such as the family home or residential care.
- Nurses and other professionals on such wards do not usually have the training or skills to meet the needs of the person's intellectual disability.
- They might expect each patient on the ward to quickly learn appropriate routines such as meal times, times for medication rounds, days of ward rounds, days when occupational therapy activities are available and so on.
- A person with ID may have poor literacy skills and lack a sense of time.
- The staff on the wards may be too busy with unpredictable acute emergencies to have time to help people with ID adjust to being in a new environment.

As a result of this lack of individualised care and attention, people with ID may feel confused or distressed. More importantly, they may feel more vulnerable in general adult ward settings, and many may be prone to abuse or exploitation.

Services have therefore argued for more collaborative working models for people with ID who have mental health needs. A recent study (Bhaumik *et al*, 2008) stresses the need for close collaboration between mainstream mental health and specialist service providers to improve the experiences of people with ID. It also stresses the importance of a clear pathway for people with ID and mental health problems, to ease the transfer between specialist and generic mental health services, and the importance of a protocol for joint working where input from both services is required.

In order to improve access to mainstream mental health services, the Green Light Toolkit (GLT) (Foundation for People with Learning Disabilities, 2004) was introduced with the aim of measuring how the *National Service Framework for Mental Health* (DH, 1999) is being implemented for people with ID in England. This audit tool provides standards that local mainstream mental health and specialist ID services, in collaboration with key stakeholders, can measure their services against using a 'traffic light' scoring system. It also provides guidance on how services can be improved and covers areas such as local partnerships, planning, accessing services, care planning, workforce planning and diversity. It can be a useful tool for services, helping them to identify gaps in their service for meeting the mental health needs of people with ID, and helping them to plan and develop a service strategy. However, very little is published about the use of the GLT and its impact on service development.

The development of an inclusive mainstream mental health service will consist of a number of factors, which should be allowed to grow and flourish over a period of time so that its effectiveness can be closely monitored. It is difficult to provide an exhaustive list, but the key factors that are needed are as follows:

- user and carer involvement in the development of services and their functioning
- effective communication systems at all levels of the service
- accessible information for people with ID, their carers and other professionals, about the types and nature of services and the therapeutic interventions offered
- a clear vision in the service of the requirements of people with ID and mental health needs, and how they can address these requirements
- appropriately trained and qualified professionals who are confident and competent to address the challenging issues of assessment and intervention

- joint training of learning disability and mental health nurses
- multi-professional education/training programmes for all professionals working in this area.

The new mental health strategy, *No Health Without Mental Health* (DH, 2011), sets out the coalition government's ambition to put mental health in the mainstream and to establish parity of esteem between services for people with mental health problems and those with physical health problems. This strategy outlines six broad principles.

1. More people of all ages and backgrounds will have better well-being and good mental health. Fewer people will develop mental health problems – by starting well, developing well, working well, living well and ageing well.

2. More people who develop mental health problems will have a good quality of life, including a greater ability to manage their own lives, stronger social relationships, a greater sense of purpose, the skills they need for living and working, improved chances in education, better employment rates and a suitable and stable place to live.

3. Fewer people with mental health problems will die prematurely, and more people with physical ill health will have better mental health.

4. Care and support, wherever it takes place, should offer access to timely, evidence-based interventions and approaches that give people the greatest choice and control over their own lives, in the least restrictive environment, and should ensure that people's human rights are protected.

5. People receiving care and support should have confidence that the services they use are of the highest quality and are at least as safe as any other public service.

6. Public understanding of mental health will improve and, as a result, negative attitudes and behaviours towards people with mental health problems will decrease.

(DH, 2011, p6)

This policy is relevant to everyone, from children and young people to those of working age and older. The mental health of people with ID is also specifically mentioned in this document, and it highlights two key aspects for the improvement of mental health services for this population and for people with autism:

- *'inclusivity of mainstream mental health services for people with learning disabilities who have mental health problems'*
- *'development of appropriate skills and provision of adjustments to meet the individual needs of people with learning disabilities and autism (recognising the increased risks of a range of physical and mental health problems for this group).'*

(DH, 2011)

Access to psychological therapies

People with ID experience severe health inequalities in terms of access to and use of appropriate therapeutic services, and recent evidence highlights continuing discrimination in receiving adequate health interventions from mainstream health services. A national newspaper in the UK reported that, *'the National Health Service is accused of causing or contributing to the deaths of at least 74 patients with a learning disability because of poor care that reveals enduring "institutional discrimination" among doctors and nurses'* (Bawden & Campbell, 2012). This discriminatory attitude has been a major topic of discussion over the last five years, and a number enquires and reports published have argued for 'reasonable adjustments' to be made by services for people with ID. As to how these adjustments work is to be monitored and evaluated over the next few years, when we might have reasonable evidence of its implementation.

The National Institute for Health and Clinical Excellence (NICE) guidelines on anxiety and depression (NICE, 2007; 2009) recommend a range of therapeutic approaches to treat people with anxiety and depression, and access to psychological therapies is a major component of the recommended interventions.

Improving access to psychological therapies (IAPT) is a major initiative for people with mental health needs. For many people with ID, however, this initiative is not fully implemented and it is not able to evaluate the effectiveness of applying the most common psychological therapies to this population. According to IAPT, the key barriers in accessing psychological therapies for people with ID include:

- professionals' lack of confidence in working with people with ID
- professionals' concerns about their ability to build a therapeutic relationship with a person with ID

- professionals' consider that psychological therapies would be better used on people with greater cognitive abilities.

(IAPT, 2009)

The positive practice guide for IAPT (IAPT, 2009) highlights the need for proper and effective engagement with people with ID, and it recommends:

- monitoring uptake of IAPT services by people with ID
- identifying the successful and unsuccessful referral pathways
- recognising that community learning disability team staff, support staff, family members, carers and advocates can all play an important role in identifying mental health problems in people with ID, and that they should be a key part of the referral pathway into the IAPT service
- recognising that people with ID themselves may be a potential resource to the IAPT service (eg. as volunteers or paid workers, including playing a part in recruiting staff)
- advertising psychological therapies in ways that are accessible and meaningful to people with ID, such as providing leaflets or audio/DVDs in easy-to-understand formats
- commissioning local voluntary sector and advocacy groups specialising in ID to raise awareness and to support people with ID to access IAPT services.

The evidence base for many psychological and other interventions for people with ID is limited, which calls for more practice-based evidence models that may help to highlight the factors contributing to the long-term sustainability of these interventions. Person-centred approaches to care and intervention are multi-dimensional as they involve family carers, teachers, frontline support workers and range of health and social care professionals. For example, a person with ID living in a supported group home may receive help and support from frontline staff and a range of professionals such as nurses, psychologists and psychiatrists. This may involve anxiety management when at home, at work, or when shopping or engaging in any social or leisure pursuits. While providing this person-centred approach, it is important for health and social care professionals to identify and record all the intricate processes involved. This detailed and careful documentation of the nature and experiences of the user, carers and professionals will help to build a rich and valid picture of the much-needed practice-based evidence for working with people with ID and mental health needs.

Disablism, risk and resilience

Disablism

The Demos Report (2004), *Disablism: How to tackle the last prejudice*, was intended to put the word 'disablism' in the context of the political and social agenda, alongside racism and sexism. It defines disablism as *'discriminatory, oppressive or abusive behaviour arising from the belief that disabled people are inferior to others'*. Emerson (2010) argues that disablism contributes to poor health outcomes for people with ID, and in a major study using secondary data to explore the possible impact of exposure to discrimination in everyday life on the health status of people with ID, he highlights that exposure to overt acts of disablism contributes to the health inequalities experienced by this population. Emerson concludes that health and social policies aimed at reducing health inequalities are likely to be more effective if they are specifically tailored to the social and cultural experiences of high-risk groups such as those with ID.

People with ID have a multiplicity of health and social care needs that require specialist help and support. O'Hara (2010) argues that, *'people with ID have a constellation of negative health determinants, including minimal education, low income, unemployment and poorly developed social networks, which are risk factors in their own right for poorer health outcome'*. Moreover, people with ID from minority ethnic communities experience exclusion and discrimination in terms of accessing and using health and social care services (Raghavan *et al*, 2009).

Risk

ID is a 'risk factor' that increases the likelihood of adverse outcomes, but it cannot predict future behaviour in itself. A combination of factors – personal, familial and social – determine whether individuals with ID will have successful academic, social and employment outcomes (Cosden *et al*, 1999). Nevertheless, people with ID are at a greater risk of developing mental health problems and being exposed to social disadvantage than their non-disabled peers (Emerson & Hatton, 2007), and they often experience serious intra- and interpersonal problems such as loneliness and depression, which can exacerbate the challenges presented by the intellectual disability itself (Cosden *et al*, 1999).

However, focused interventions in building resilience can provide people with ID with a buffer against these negative experiences, and Emerson and Hatton (2007) suggests that building the resilience of children with ID and their families can help reduce the personal, social and economic costs associated with mental health disorders.

Resilience

Resilience is the term used to refer to the maintenance of positive adaptation by individuals within the context of significant adversity (Luthar & Cicchetti, 2000). It is a dynamic process involving interactions between various risks and protective processes, both internal and external to the individual, that act to mitigate the influences of adverse life events (Margalit, 2003). It encompasses three areas:

- individual characteristics
- their families
- the societies in which they live.

In societal terms, the most important influences are those of school and the broader social environment. Given that it involves an interaction between the person and their social and physical ecology, resilience is always contextual and can be achieved in a variety of ways across contexts and cultures (Didkowsky *et al*, 2010).

The resilience model shifts focus away from deficits, looking instead at the strengths in individuals and systems, and is therefore more useful for educators and therapists. It is also useful from policy and practice perspectives since it can help to inform guidance on prevention and intervention efforts (Murray, 2003). By identifying what it is that makes some people resilient, it should be possible to foster those skills in those who are less so. While the resilience of non-disabled individuals who have been exposed to severe adversity has been widely researched (Howard *et al*, 1999), this has not been matched by research into the ways individuals with ID construct resilience for themselves.

Resilience-building activities should be carefully linked to the types and range of interventions offered and their effectiveness in building emotional well-being in people with ID. Luther and Cicchetti (2000) provide a set of guiding principles that are very relevant to people with ID:

- interventions must have a strong basis in theory and research of the particular group
- efforts should be directed not only toward the reduction of negative

outcomes or maladjustment among targeted groups, but also toward the promotion of dimensions of positive adaptation or competence

■ interventions must be designed not only to reduce negative influences (vulnerability factors) but also to capitalise on specific resources within particular populations

■ interventions should target salient vulnerability and protective processes that operate across multiple levels of influence (influences stemming from the community, family as well as from the individual)

■ interventions should have a strong developmental focus

■ the contextual relevance of the overall intervention aims, as well as of the specific intervention strategies, must be ensured

■ intervention efforts should aim at fostering services that can eventually become self-sustaining

■ wherever possible, data from interventions groups should be compared with those of appropriate comparison groups

■ there must be careful documentation and evaluation of the interventions (of all the gains and unanticipated problems).

Conclusion

Enabling people with ID to develop emotional well-being is both an art and a science. It is an art because of the diverse roles that professionals and carers have to play when engaging with people with ID. Experienced professionals should reflect on their work with a person with ID and, through publications, provide stories of the art of implementing such interventions. These stories will highlight the processes and the complexity of implementing and evaluating some of the much needed psychological interventions for people with ID. We should not limit the exploration and use of psychological and other appropriate intervention strategies for this population because of the lack of evidence base. Imagination is a key asset here, as it helps to explore and combine a range of methodologies and approaches that can be implemented easily and cost effectively. This will undoubtedly help the advancement of professional practice and contribute to the development of evidence based on practice models. As Albert Einstein once said, *'Imagination is more important than knowledge. Knowledge is limited. Imagination encircles the world.'*

Summary

■ Providing services for people with ID with additional mental health needs is a challenge for services. Health and social policy directives identify the gaps in our mainstream mental health services and identify the need to provide appropriate therapeutic services for people with ID with mental health needs.

■ Access to psychological therapies for people with ID need to be fully explored and appropriate modifications and adaptations should be made.

■ Building resilience is of paramount importance in enabling and empowering people with ID with additional mental health needs.

References

Bawden A & Campbell D (2012) NHS accused over deaths of disabled patients. *The Guardian* **2 January**.

Bhaumik S, Tyrer F, McGrowther C & Gangadharan S (2008) Psychiatric service use and psychiatric disorders in adults with intellectual disability. *Journal of Intellectual Disability Research* **52** (11) 986–995.

Cosden M, Elliott K, Sharon N & Kelemen E (1999) Self-understanding and self-esteem in children with learning disabilities. *Learning Disability Quarterly* **22** (4) 279–290.

Demos (2004) *Disablism: How to tackle the last prejudice*. London: Demos. Available at: http://www.demos.co.uk/publications/disablism.

Department of Health (1999) *National Service Framework for Mental Health: Modern standards and service models*. London: Department of Health.

Department of Health (2001) *Valuing People: A new strategy for learning disability for the 21st century*. London: TSO.

Department of Health (2009) *Valuing People Now: A three year strategy for people with learning disabilities*. London: Department of Health.

Department of Health (2011) *No Health Without Mental health: A cross government mental health outcome strategy for people of all ages*. London: Department of Health.

Didkowsky N, Ungar M & Liebenberg L (2010) Using visual methods to capture embedded processes of resilience for youth across cultures and contexts. *Journal of the Canadian Academy of Child and Adolescent Psychiatry* **19** (1) 12–18.

Dosen A (1993) Mental health and mental illness in persons with retardation: what are we talking about? In: R Fletcher and A Dosen (Eds) *Mental Health Aspects of Mental Retardation*. New York: Lexington Books.

Emerson E (2001) *Challenging Behaviour: Analysis and intervention in people with severe intellectual disabilities*. Cambridge: Cambridge University Press.

Emerson E (2010) Self-reported exposure to disablism is associated with poorer self-reported health and well-being among adults with intellectual disabilities in England: A cross-sectional survey. *Public Health* **124** (12) 682–689.

Emerson E & Hatton C (2007) Mental health of children and adolescents with intellectual disabilities in Britain. *The British Journal of Psychiatry* **191** (6) 493–499.

Foundation for People with Learning Disabilities (2004) *The Green Light for Mental Health: How good are your mental health services for people with learning disabilities?* London: Foundation for People with Learning Disabilities.

Howard S, Dryden J & Johnson B (1999) Childhood resilience: review and critique of literature. *Oxford Review of Education* **25** (3) 307–323.

Improving Access to Psychological Therapies (IAPT) (2009) *Learning Disabilities: Positive practice guide*. London: Department of Health.

Luther S & Cicchetti D (2000) The construct of resilience implications for interventions and social policies. *Developmental Psychopathology* **12** (4) 857–885.

Margalit M (2003) Resilience model among individuals with learning disabilities: proximal and distal influences. *Learning Disabilities Research & Practice* **18** (2) 82–86.

Miller M (2002) Resilience elements in students with learning disabilities. *Journal of Clinical Psychology* **58** (3) 291–298.

Moss S, Emerson E, Kiernan C, Turner S, Hatton C & Atborz A (2000) Psychiatric symptoms in adults with learning disability and challenging behaviour. *The British Journal of Psychiatry* **177** 452–456.

Moss S, Prosser H, Costello H, Simpson N, Patel P, Rowe S, Turner S & Hatton C (1998) Reliability and validity the PAS-ADD checklist for detecting disorders in adults with intellectual disability *Journal of Intellectual Disability Research* **42** (2) 173–183.

Murray C (2003) Risk factors, protective factors, vulnerability and resilience. *Remedial and Special Education* **24** (1) 16–26.

National Institute of Health and Clinical Excellence (2007) *Anxiety: Management of anxiety.* London: NICE.

National Institute of Health and Clinical Excellence (2009) *Depression: The treatment and management of depression in adults*. London: NICE.

O'Hara J (2010) Health care and intellectual disability. In: J O'Hara, J McCarthy and N Bouras (Eds) *Intellectual Disability and Ill Health: A review of evidence*. Cambridge: Cambridge University Press.

Raghavan R, Newell R, Waseem F & Small N (2009) A randomised controlled trial of a specialist liaison worker model for young people with intellectual disabilities with behaviour and mental health needs. *Journal of Applied Research in Intellectual Disabilities* **22** 256–263.

Chapter 2

Anxiety disorders in people with intellectual disabilities

Tonye Sikabofori and Anupama Iyer

Overview

This chapter provides an overview of the manifestations of anxiety disorders in people with ID and describes the presentation of these disorders in the general population, as well as the difficulties in recognising and assessing them in persons with ID. It also explains the developmental antecedents and risk factors for the disorders.

Learning objectives

- To understand the phenomenology of anxiety disorders.
- To understand their presentation in persons with ID.
- To understand the developmental trajectory, co-morbidity and risk factors.
- To review the assessment instruments for anxiety disorders in people with ID.

Introduction

The history of recognised anxiety disorders in people with ID is a relatively recent and chequered one, and one that has gone full circle from doubts about its very existence to the increasing recognition that it may be as common, if not more common, in people with ID than the general population (Deb *et al*, 2001; Bailey & Andrews, 2003). The recognition and management of anxiety disorders presents unique challenges in people with ID, and there are several considerations with regards to phenomenology, confounders and co-morbidity that are unique to this population. This chapter will discuss these issues in detail.

The nature of anxiety

Anxiety is a fundamental human emotion with its evolutionary foundations in enabling an optimal assessment of threats to survival. Fear is an allied negative affective state, which is elicited when a person confronts an immediate threat or danger. Anxiety therefore differs from fear in being a reaction to impending but not immediately present danger. Its anticipatory nature defines it, and while this anticipatory quality enhances performance when optimal, it can impair performance when excessive (The Yerkes-Dodson Law (Yerkes & Dodson, 1908)).

Anxiety has psychological, physiological and behavioural concomitants:

- The psychological effects are characterised by 'feelings of dysphoria' (American Psychiatric Association, 2000).
- The physiological concomitants include symptoms related to hyper-arousal, such as dry mouth, breathlessness, increased heart rate and tremulousness.
- Anxiety may be manifested in a range of behaviours, from agitation and aggression through to avoidance.

These cognitive, physiological and behavioural concomitants carry different weights and may be variably critical in establishing a diagnosis of anxiety disorder in different populations. For instance, it has been suggested that children may experience the somatic (or physiological) symptoms of panic disorder, but lack the cognitive ability to attribute these sensations to internal factors (Nelles & Barlow, 1988). Similarly, people with more severe ID may manifest with the behaviour concomitants alone without the subjective cognitive states (Matson *et al*, 1997).

Anxiety disorders represent an extreme in the continuum of responses to adversity and perceived threats, and become pathological when they are relatively pervasive, long-standing and result in impairments to adaptive function and lead to significant distress.

Types of anxiety disorders

Generalised anxiety disorder

Generalised anxiety disorder (GAD) presents as a persistent anxiety without the specific symptoms that characterise phobic anxiety disorder or panic disorder. It is subjective apprehension, worry or fear, with motor tension, autonomic hyperactivity, vigilance and scanning. A person with ID might complain of feeling 'on the edge', with interrupted sleep patterns or difficulty sleeping, alongside fatigue on waking.

The essential feature is anxiety that is generalised and persistent but not restricted to, or even strongly predominating in, any particular environmental circumstances (ie. it is 'free floating'). As in other anxiety disorders, the dominant symptoms are highly variable, but complaints of continuous feelings of nervousness, trembling, muscular tension, sweating, light-headedness, palpitations, dizziness and epigastric discomfort are common. Fears that the individual or a relative will become ill or have an accident are often expressed, together with a variety of other worries. This disorder is more common in women, and often related to chronic environmental stress. Its course is variable but tends to be fluctuating and chronic.

Panic disorder

The essential features of panic disorder are recurrent attacks of severe anxiety (panic) that are not restricted to any particular situation or set of circumstances, and which are therefore unpredictable. As in other anxiety disorders, the dominant symptoms vary from person to person, but the sudden onset of palpitations, chest pain, choking sensations, dizziness, and feelings of unreality (depersonalisation or derealisation) are common. There is also, almost invariably, a secondary fear of dying, losing control or going mad. Individual attacks usually last for minutes only, though sometimes longer – their frequency and the course of the disorder are both rather variable. An individual experiencing a panic attack often experiences a crescendo of fear and autonomic symptoms, which results in an exit, usually hurried, from wherever they may be. If this occurs in a specific situation, such as on a bus or in a crowd, the patient may subsequently avoid that situation. Similarly, frequent and unpredictable panic attacks produce fear of being alone or going into public places. A panic attack is often followed by a persistent fear of having another attack. For a definite diagnosis, several severe attacks of autonomic anxiety should have occurred within a period of about one month.

Agoraphobia

Agoraphobia is seen strictly as a fear of open spaces and it accounts for about 60% of phobic patients seen by psychiatrists. It has a fluctuating course once it is established and it may persist for years. Agoraphobia is usually an anxiety of, and therefore avoidance of, places or situations from which escape could be embarrassing or difficult, and in which help may not be available in the event of a panic attack or its symptoms. Most individuals with agoraphobia are women and the onset is usually early in adult life. Depressive and obsessional symptoms and social phobias may also be present but do not dominate the clinical picture. In the absence of effective treatment, agoraphobia often becomes chronic, often with a fluctuating course over time.

Case study: Mr P

Mr P is a 24 year old with severe ID and fragile X syndrome (see p30). While having a trip in the car around the local area he became distressed and agitated and physically attacked his paid carer. The police were called to support and move him to the local psychiatric hospital, where he presented as calm and appropriate in his behaviour.

Mr P was initially unable to give an account of his earlier distress. According to his care giver, who observed his symptoms and behaviour, he had had a two-year history of becoming nervous in certain situations, for example while travelling in a car for long journeys. The paid care giver and staff from the residential home described how Mr P would worry about being involved in an accident and have symptoms such as sweating, shaking and breathing very fast. He had also been seen to hold his chest as if in pain.

Collateral history obtained from the staff at the residential home indicated that the onset of his anxiety symptoms correlated with a number of bereavements of significant people in his life, including the death of his parents in an accident that he witnessed.

Continued >

However, Mr P had become so nervous in social situations that he had been living an extremely restricted lifestyle, avoiding situations that involved travelling in a car to activities. There were no biological features of a mood disorder.

After observations, the local learning disability psychiatric team made a diagnosis of panic disorder with agoraphobia. A medication (selective serotonin re-uptake inhibitor) was prescribed along with psychological treatment for anxiety disorder. He engaged well with the treatment programme and after six months his activities in the community increased, which he enjoyed.

Panic disorder without agoraphobia is usually characterised by unexpected recurrent panic attacks for which there is a persistent concern. The other is panic disorder with agoraphobia, such as in the example above, which is characterised both by recurrent unexpected panic attacks and agoraphobia. There are other situations where agoraphobia without a history of panic disorder can occur, and this is basically the presence of agoraphobia with panic-type symptoms, but without a history of unexpected panic attacks.

Social phobia

Social phobia often starts in adolescence and is centred on a fear of being scrutinised by other people in comparatively small groups (as opposed to crowds), leading to avoidance of social situations. Unlike most other phobias, social phobias are equally common in men and women. They may be discrete (ie. restricted to eating in public, to public speaking, or to encounters with the opposite sex) or diffuse, involving almost all social situations outside the family circle. A fear of vomiting in public may be important. Social phobias are usually associated with low self-esteem and fear of criticism. They may present as a complaint of blushing, hand tremors, nausea or an urgent need to urinate, and the individual is sometimes convinced that one of these secondary manifestations of anxiety is the primary problem. Symptoms may progress to panic attacks. Avoidance is often notable, and in extreme cases may result in almost complete social isolation.

All of the following criteria should be fulfilled for a definite diagnosis of social phobia.

1. Psychological or autonomic symptoms must primarily be manifestations of anxiety and not secondary to other symptoms, such as delusions or obsessional thoughts.

2. Anxiety must be restricted to (or occur mainly in) at least two of the following situations: crowds, public places, travelling away from home, travelling alone.

3. Avoidance of the phobic situation must be, or have been, a prominent feature.

Specific (isolated) phobias

These are phobias restricted to highly specific situations such as fears of particular animals, heights, thunder, darkness, flying, closed spaces, urinating or defecating in public toilets, eating certain foods, dentistry, the sight of blood or injury, or the fear of exposure to specific diseases. Although the triggering situation is discrete, contact with it can evoke panic as in agoraphobia or social phobias. Specific phobias usually arise in childhood or early adult life and can persist for decades if they remain untreated. The seriousness of the resulting handicap depends on how easy it is for the person to avoid the phobic situation. Fear of the phobic situation tends not to fluctuate, in contrast to agoraphobia.

Specific phobia becomes clinically significant when there is exposure to a specific feared object or situation that then leads to an avoidance behaviour. It is characterised by a persistent irrational fear of, and compelling desire to avoid, situations in which the person may be exposed to the scrutiny of others. A person may also present with a fear where they behave in a manner that is humiliating or embarrassing for them (eg. blushing, vomiting or shaking).

Illness phobia is a persistent and intense fear of illness, focused on specific disorders such as heart disease or cancer, or an intense fear of death and dying. Radiation sickness and sexually transmitted infections, including more recently AIDS, are also common subjects of disease phobias. There are usually chronic ruminations but no apparent attempt at resistance. A previous illness in an individual, or a relative or carer, may therefore act as a precipitant. There may also be associated mental disorders such as depression.

Obsessive compulsive disorder

The essential feature of obsessive compulsive disorder (OCD) is the presence of recurrent obsessional thoughts or compulsive acts. (For brevity, 'obsessional' will be used subsequently in place of 'obsessive compulsive' when referring to symptoms.) Obsessional thoughts are ideas, images or impulses that enter the individual's mind again and again in a stereotyped form. They are almost invariably distressing (because they are violent or obscene, or simply because they are perceived as senseless) and the person often tries, unsuccessfully, to resist them. They are, however, recognised as the individual's own thoughts, even though they are involuntary and often repugnant. Compulsive acts or rituals are stereotyped behaviours that are repeated again and again. They are not inherently enjoyable, nor do they result in the completion of inherently useful tasks. The individual often views them as preventing some objectively unlikely event, often involving harm to, or caused by, the individual.

Usually, although not invariably, the individual recognises this behaviour as pointless or ineffectual and, as mentioned, repeated attempts are made to resist it, but in very long-standing cases this resistance may be minimal. Autonomic anxiety symptoms are often present, but distressing feelings of internal or psychological tension without obvious autonomic arousal are also common. There is a close relationship between obsessional symptoms, particularly obsessional thoughts, and depression. Individuals with OCD often have depressive symptoms, and patients with a recurrent depressive disorder may develop obsessional thoughts during episodes of depression. In either situation, increases or decreases in the severity of the depressive symptoms are generally accompanied by parallel changes in the severity of the obsessional symptoms.

OCD is equally common in men and women, and there are often prominent compulsive features in the underlying personality. Onset is usually in childhood or early adult life, and the course is variable and more likely to be chronic in the absence of significant depressive symptoms.

For a definite diagnosis, obsessional symptoms or compulsive acts, or both, must be present on most days for at least two successive weeks, and be a source of distress or must interfere with activities. The obsessional symptoms should have the following characteristics:

■ they must be recognised as the individual's own thoughts or impulses

- there must be at least one thought or act that is still resisted unsuccessfully, even though others may be present that the person no longer resists
- the thought of carrying out the act must not in itself be pleasurable (simple relief of tension or anxiety is not regarded as pleasure in this sense)
- the thoughts, images or impulses must be unpleasantly repetitive.

Case study: John

John is a 27-year-old man with mild ID who works at a supermarket. He has a compulsive need to wash his hands and a fear of contamination by germs. John has to wear gloves when he is at work and he has rituals surrounding what he will touch and what he will avoid. When washing his hands, he will first dig his nails into the soap bar and then wash his hands without touching the sink or taps. He would not use a towel to dry his hands, instead he using paper towels. His obsessional symptoms are affecting his work. In the past he had rituals whereby he had to wash his face in a certain way. This seems to have improved over time. Clinically, the diagnosis appears to be OCD.

Post-traumatic stress disorder

Post-traumatic stress disorder (PTSD) arises as a delayed and/or protracted response to a stressful event or situation (either of short or long duration) that is exceptionally threatening or catastrophic in nature, and which is likely to cause pervasive distress in almost anyone (eg. natural or manmade disasters, combat, serious accident, witnessing the violent death of others, or being the victim of torture, terrorism, rape or other serious crimes). Predisposing factors such as personality traits (eg. compulsive, asthenic) or a previous history of neurotic illness may lower the threshold for the development of the syndrome or aggravate its course, but they are neither necessary nor sufficient to explain its occurrence.

Typical symptoms include episodes of repeatedly reliving the trauma in intrusive memories ('flashbacks') or dreams, occurring against a persistent background of a sense of emotional 'numbness', detachment from other people, unresponsiveness to surroundings, anhedonia (loss of pleasure or interest in activities) and avoidance of activities and situations reminiscent of the trauma. Rarely, there may be dramatic and acute bursts of fear, panic or aggression, triggered by stimuli arousing a sudden recollection and/or re-enactment of the trauma or of the original reaction to it.

There is usually a state of autonomic hyperarousal with hypervigilance (an enhanced startle reaction) and insomnia. Anxiety and depression are commonly associated with the above symptoms and signs, and suicidal thoughts are not infrequent. Excessive use of alcohol or drugs may be a complicating factor. According to the International Classification of Diseases (ICD-10) (WHO, 2010) criteria, the onset follows the trauma with a latency period that may range from a few weeks to a number of months (but rarely exceeding six months). The course is fluctuating but recovery can be expected in the majority of cases. In a small proportion of patients the condition may show a chronic course over many years and a transition to an enduring personality change.

PTSD should not generally be diagnosed unless there is evidence that it arose within six months of a traumatic event of exceptional severity. A 'probable' diagnosis might still be possible if the delay between the event and the onset was longer than six months, provided that the clinical manifestations are typical and no alternative identification of the disorder is plausible (eg. anxiety, OCD or a depressive episode). In addition to evidence of trauma, there must be a repetitive, intrusive recollection or re-enactment of the event in memories, daytime imagery or dreams. Conspicuous emotional detachment, a numbness of feeling and avoidance of stimuli that might arouse recollection of the trauma are often present but are not essential for the diagnosis. The autonomic disturbances, mood disorder and behavioural abnormalities all contribute to the diagnosis but are not of prime importance.

Other forms of anxiety disorder

Acute stress disorder presents quite similar to PTSD, but the features occur in the immediate aftermath of an extremely traumatic event. Anxiety disorder due to a general medical condition is a direct physiological consequence of a general medical condition. Substance induced anxiety disorder is, as the name suggests, a direct physiological consequence of a medication or toxin exposure, including drug abuse. Anxiety disorder not otherwise specified was introduced to distinguish anxiety disorders that have prominent anxiety or phobic avoidance but basically do not meet the criteria for any of the specific anxiety disorders described previously.

Behaviour phenotypes

The term 'behaviour phenotype' was introduced by Nyhan (1972) to describe particular behaviours that are integrally associated with specific genetic syndromes. Behaviour phenotypes are of particular interest when it is possible to use the phenotypic features to locate a gene of interest by deletion mapping (Skuse, 2000). Anxiety disorders have been described as occurring in a wide variety genetic disorders.

Fragile X syndrome (FXS). This is the most common inherited cause of mental retardation. The behaviour phenotype of FXS includes hyperarousal, hyperactivity, aggression, anxiety and extreme sensitivity to sensory stimuli (Hagerman, 1996). Avoidance behaviours during greetings, such as turning the eyes and body away while shaking hands (Wolff *et al*, 1989) have been described as characteristic of fragile X phenotype, and Bregman *et al* (1988) suggest that the poor eye contact in FXS relates to anxiety rather than being related to autistic deficits.

Fragile X subjects regularly present with significant degrees of expressed anxiety, including persistent worry regarding competence, performance and social acceptability, apprehension of future events, marked self-consciousness and physical complaints without physical basis (Bregman *et al*, 1988). The carriers of the fragile X premutation have a notably high lifetime risk of mood and anxiety disorders (Bourgeois *et al*, 2011).

Prader-Willi syndrome. Dykens *et al* (1996) reported a high incidence of OCD in association with Prader-Willi syndrome, and it has been postulated that the compulsive behaviours in Prader-Willi syndrome are similar to compulsions seen in children without developmental disabilities. There are very few obsessional thoughts reported, however, and the range of compulsive symptoms is relatively restricted (Clarke *et al*, 2002).

William's syndrome. William's syndrome is caused by a micro deletion on one of the chromosome 7s and affects about one in 20,000 people. Fears and phobias are salient manifestations of anxiety in people with William's syndrome, and they are more likely to have specific phobias compared to those with other anxiety disorders. Various hypotheses have been put forward to account for this increase, for instance that high rates of fears or phobias may be associated with specific genetic or biological vulnerabilities that interact with life experiences and with certain aspects of the William's syndrome phenotype. Fears of falling from high places, for example, may relate to the joint contractures and problems with gross motor co-ordination balance. Fears of loud sounds such as thunderstorms and sirens may be related to hyperacusis (Dykens, 2003).

Epidemiology

Anxiety disorders have been shown to produce disproportionate morbidity, functional impairment and increased use of healthcare services. They have a four to seven per cent prevalence rate in the normal population, accounting for 27% of psychiatric consultations in general practice and 80% of psychiatric outpatients. It is also reported that women are more affected than men, with females having higher rates of all types of anxiety disorders than males. However, this gender bias has not been replicated in studies of people with ID (Cooper *et al*, 2007). The National Psychiatric Morbidity Survey (National Centre for Social Research, 1997) showed a point prevalence of any neurotic disorder to be 19.5% in females and 17.3% in males, while for GAD the split was 3.4% female and 2.8% male. For phobia-related anxiety, the prevalence was 1.4% for females and 0.7% for males, and for panic disorder it was 0.9% and 0.8% respectively.

As already mentioned, some studies have suggested that there is a higher prevalence of anxiety disorders in adults with ID than in the general population (Deb *et al*, 2001; Bailey & Andrews, 2003). This may be due to several reasons, including low self-esteem, inadequate ability to express distress, decreased adaptive abilities and insufficient coping strategies. Kessler *et al* (1994) demonstrated that all types of mental disorder and illnesses, including anxiety disorders, decline with increasing educational status. It therefore follows that people with ID are more likely to have some form of anxiety disorder, and over protection and limited linguistic skills may lead to greater difficulties in elaborating and reasoning away fears (Pickersgill *et al*, 1994). There is also evidence that people with ID are more vulnerable to stressful life events, having poorer coping skills. Lifetime adversity and a lack of adequate social support can also trigger an anxiety disorder.

Lund (1988) found neurotic traits in 25 out of 44 adults (57%), but when diagnostic criteria were used, none were found to have a neurosis. Myers and Pueschel (1991) also found that five of 497 people (one per cent) with Down's syndrome had a phobic disorder. The prevalence rates of psychiatric disorders in adults with Down's syndrome are similar to rates in people without Down's syndrome but with ID, although these are increased compared with the general population.

Cooper (1997) identified a random sample of 81 individuals aged 20 to 64 years, and everyone over 64 from the Leicestershire Learning Disability Register, giving a total sample size of 270. All of the participants underwent clinical assessment and were diagnosed according to the ICD-10 (WHO, 2010) diagnostic criteria. Cooper found a lifetime prevalence for all psychiatric disorders of 49.2%, including possible dementia, Rhett's syndrome and problem behaviour.

Cooper also found the prevalence of OCD in people with ID to be 2.5%, which is higher than the general population, GAD and specific phobia to be six per cent, and agoraphobia to be 1.5%. Obsessional thoughts are hard for people with ID to describe. Compulsions, on the other hand, are easily observed, but this is quite difficult to distinguish from stereotypes, tics and autism. Raghavan (1997) conducted a literature review that found higher rates of anxiety disorders in people with ID.

Co-morbidity is also a significant problem, and Kessler *et al* (1994) reported that about 75% of individuals with anxiety disorder met the criteria for at least one co-morbid psychiatric disorder. While Bailey and Andrews (2003) described that people with ID and anxiety disorders are well recognised, Reiss *et al* (1982) highlighted that they may be under reported and undiagnosed (Verhoeven & Tuinier, 1997).

From the few studies above, it is evident that anxiety disorders are at least as common among people with ID as they are among the general population, and probably more so.

Developmental perspective

Mild fears are common among children and adolescents (Silverman & Nelles, 1990), but anxiety disorders remain among the most common form of childhood psychopathology (Bernstein & Borchardt, 1991). Composite conclusions from a number of prevalent studies indicate that 20% of young people have one of the anxiety disorders, and over 50% have functional impairments affecting social and educational functioning in the general population.

There is growing evidence for anxiety disorders emerging early in childhood, and they may be among disorders with the earliest onset, being present in children younger than 12 (Merikangas & Kalaydjian, 2009).

There is also growing evidence that anxiety disorders during the lifespan have developmental antecedents in early life (Pine, 2009). Early onset anxiety disorders may also represent the start of a developmental trajectory towards externalising and mood disorders, and may be childhood precursors to adult anxiety disorders.

Developmental consequences may be affected both by constitutional traits inherent to individuals and by environmental influences. For example, a parental history of anxiety, in particular, co-aggregates with anxiety disorders in young people (Pine, 2009). One of the earliest temperamental traits predisposing a vulnerability to anxiety disorders has been called behavioural inhibition, which is characterised by increased physiological reactivity and behavioural withdrawal in the face of new stimuli or challenging situations. Another trait marker for anxiety disorder is 'anxiety sensitivity', which is characterised by the belief that anxiety sensations are indicative of harmful physiological and social consequences (Pine, 2009).

The most common disorder in childhood is specific phobia, followed by social phobia and GAD. The peak ages for the onset of these different disorders varies, with panic disorder being rare in children under 12 and separation anxiety disorder being most common in pre-pubertal children (Kashani & Orvaschel, 1990; Merkangas & Kalaydjian, 2009). Over-anxious disorder, meanwhile, is common in late childhood, social phobias become more common in late adolescence, and GAD and OCD have a later age of onset.

There are a few robust studies specifically on the prevalence of anxiety disorders in young people with ID. However, Dekker and Koot (2003) is one such study, and it reported a prevalence of anxiety disorder of 21.9% (based on parental ratings on the Diagnostic Interview Schedule for Children). Emerson (2003), meanwhile, reported significantly higher rates of anxiety disorder among a cohort of young people with ID compared to their non-disabled peers.

Anxiety disorders in individuals with pervasive developmental disorders

It is common for people with pervasive developmental disorders, such as those on the autistic spectrum, to display anxiety in social settings, which could be due to their difficulty in reciprocating social and emotional cues. These individuals become anxious, and their anxieties are more pronounced if a fixed routine or pattern is disrupted because they need predictability, and changes in their life, no matter how small, can result in significant upset (Gillott & Standen, 2007).

Repetitive behaviours and stereotypy are quite characteristic of autistic spectrum disorder, and it can sometimes be difficult to distinguish these from features or rituals exhibited by individuals with OCD. This difficulty also means that it is difficult to say if it is a source of comfort or displeasure in people with autism. Social anxiety is often displayed or is more pronounced in those with Asperger's syndrome, especially those who have high functioning autism.

Biological factors

Anxiety, as a physical response to various external and internal stimuli, is usually shaped by several systems and mechanisms, and the diversity of anxiety disorders is most likely to be as a result of differences in the function and dysfunction of these systems. The body's flight or fight response is a complex reaction to perceived danger resulting in a heightened state of arousal and a focusing of attention on the source of potential danger. This involves multiple systems including the limbic system, the pre-frontal cortex, the cerebellum and the brain nuclei. The frontal lobe is usually involved in evaluating, planning and co-ordinating strategies, as well as making decisions.

The two key regulatory centres, the hippocampus and amygdala, are the major centres in the main nuclei of the limbic system, and basically control memory and emotions. These two key areas activate the hypothalamic pituitary adrenal cortical axis, which supports the proposition of anxiety. Coplan and Lydiard (1998) described the anatomical projections between the hippocampus, amygdala and the hypothalamus. Coplan and Lydiard (1998) also demonstrated that a number of neurotransmitters are implicated in anxiety disorders, particularly feedback systems where serotonin and gamma-aminobutyric acid (GABA) function as inhibitory neurotransmitters, so a blockade of these serotonin receptors induces anxiety.

There is also an association of neurosis with a short variance of the serotonin transporter gene regulatory region and this confirms the genetic basis of trait anxiety on a molecular basis (Lesch *et al*, 1996). Neuroimaging has shown that people with PTSD have a loss of dendrites resulting in a reduction in the size of the hippocampus. McEwen (1998) reported that the loss of cells is thought to be a consequence of increases in the glucocorticoids triggered by excess stress.

Assessment dilemmas and challenges

Recognising anxiety disorder in people with ID presents unique challenges due to the presentation of the disorders, challenges in the assessment process, and specific risk factors for anxiety disorder in this population, which are different from those in the general population. Difficulties in recognition are in part due to the changeable nature of anxiety as a symptom, which presents across a range of disorders (Pine, 2009). Anxiety is also a fundamental human emotion that only becomes pathological when it has a disruptive effect on adaptive function (Bailey & Andrews, 2003).

ID in itself has a mediating effect on the diagnosis of anxiety disorders. There is a recognised tendency among people with ID to minimise the extent of their distress and disability and to adopt a 'cloak of competence' (Edgerton, 1967). The symptoms of a psychiatric disorder may also be expressed differently in people with ID than the general population. Sovner (1986) identified four such processes that may affect diagnostic consideration.

1. Baseline exaggeration: the emergent mental illness may present as an exaggeration of characteristic behaviours, for example anxiety disorders presenting as an increase in agitation or hyperactivity.

2. Intellectual distortion: difficulties in abstract thinking may also impact on the conceptualisation of the more cognitive aspects of anxiety, like apprehension and social fears.

3. Psychosocial masking: relating to the different life experiences of persons with ID, for instance limited social opportunities may mask the full expression of avoidance behaviours in someone with agoraphobia.

4. Cognitive disintegration: limited coping skills may lead to a decreased ability to withstand stress.

Diagnostic systems that rely on language-based self-reports may put people with ID at a particular disadvantage because of their inability to communicate their distress. Matson *et al* (1997) have postulated that in people with more severe ID, behavioural manifestations may be the most important indication of anxiety in the absence of a verbal account.

As already mentioned, anxiety may present as a range of non-specific behaviours such as irritability, agitation, aggression and distractibility, and it may therefore become difficult to differentiate between symptoms of an anxiety disorder and those that are assumed to be a manifestation of developmental disabilities. Symptoms may therefore be misattributed to the developmental disorder rather than an emergent mental illness. Reiss *et al* (1982) have described this phenomenon as 'diagnostic overshadowing', and Khreim and Mikkelsen (1997) emphasise that increased diagnostic weight should be given to behavioural manifestations of anxiety.

The assessment process remains a vital tool in recognising and diagnosing anxiety disorders in the absence of reliable imaging or neuro-functional markers. The assessment of anxiety disorders in persons with ID presents unique challenges in accommodating various communication and cognitive styles, and in placing greater weight on informant reports and observable behaviours in lieu of self-report (Prosser & Bromley, 1998). Basing a diagnosis on informant reports and inferring from observable behaviours creates additional filters through which the information process can be further verified (Deb & Iyer, 2004).

Informant accounts are very useful in describing observable behaviours, but they may be less useful in eliciting subjective states such as depersonalisation, and it also relies on the informant's understanding of mental illness (Borthwick-Duffy & Eynman, 1990). Furthermore, an informant may be subject to diagnostic overshadowing and also be influenced by the nature of their relationship with the person, as well as prior diagnostic considerations like challenging behaviours. However, informant accounts may have a particular role to play in establishing a timeline to life events and in identifying changes from baseline, as well as establishing any deterioration in functional abilities.

If conducting an interview with a person with ID, it may have to be specially adapted for a number of reasons:

- people with ID are more likely to have had negative experiences within medical settings
- they report a fear of doctors more than age-matched adults (Duff *et al*, 1981)
- they may have greater concerns about the consequences of the interview (Prosser & Bromley, 1998)
- assessments in unfamiliar locations may contribute to anxiety

- people with ID may have a range of communication difficulties, both receptive and expressive (Moss,1999), and a range of sensory difficulties that may impact on their participation

- their responses are particularly subject to response bias such as 'yea-saying' (Heal & Sigelman, 1995; Finlay & Lyons, 2002), compliance and 'nay-saying' (to taboo questions) (Budd *et al*, 1981)

- suggestibility may influence how diagnostic criteria are elicited in persons with ID.

Any diagnostic interviews with people with ID therefore need checks and balances built in to avoid response sets and to discourage power asymmetry (Rapley, 1995).

Good practice guidelines

1. Optimal use of setting: qualitative research suggests the use of settings familiar to clients in order to minimise anxiety (Edgerton *et al*, 1984). It may also be useful to interview clients with informants before interviewing them alone.

2. Flexible interview times: several short interviews rather than one long one may enhance engagement and minimise the disruptive effects of distractibility.

3. Use of framework statements: clear introductions and framework statements outlining the purpose of the assessment are key to minimising the person's distress.

4. Minimising response sets: Finlay and Lyons (2002) have suggested alternatives to closed questions to minimise the clients responding in an acquiescent fashion, including the use of 'either/or' questions. For example, 'do you feel OK or anxious?' instead of 'are you OK?' or 'are you anxious?'. Use of shorter sentences and limiting options has also been suggested (Wehmeyer, 1994).

5. Using pictures and symbols: using pictures and symbols minimises last option effects to verbal questions and allows for non-verbal responses such as nodding (Sigelman *et al*, 1981).

6. Clarifications and probing: gentle clarifications and sensitive probing may improve the validity of responses. The use of anchor events such as birthdays may be useful in establishing timelines regarding onset of symptoms. Summarising and re-capping key information enables clarification and minimises the effects of distractibility (Moss, 1999).

7. Informant checks: these are particularly useful in corroborating factual data and in clarifying ambiguous aspects of the client's communication.

8. Use of behavioural observation and use of information from multiple sources improves the validity of the assessment.

Adaptations to diagnostic criteria

Whether it is appropriate to use the ICD-10 (WHO, 2010) and the Diagnostic and Statistical Manual of Mental Disorders (DSM-IV-TR) (American Psychiatric Association, 2000) diagnostic systems for people with ID has been questioned. Mikkelsen and McKenna (1999), for example, have proposed that the validity of psychiatric diagnostic criteria varies inversely with the level of intelligence, both because of an increase in non-specific organic factors and the difficulty in ascertaining subjective phenomenon in people who have difficulties with language. People with ID may also present with patterns of behaviour that do not conform to the DSM-IV-TR or ICD-10 criteria for a specific mental disorder (Szymanski et al, 1998). Standard criteria may have a role to play in assessing those with mild to moderate levels of ID (Masi et al, 2002; Stavrakaki, 2002), but Matson et al (1997) concluded that only the behavioural symptoms associated with anxiety could be reliably assessed.

In response to this, the Royal College of Psychiatrists developed a diagnostic system derived from ICD-10. The Diagnostic Criteria for Psychiatric Disorders for use with Adults with Learning Disabilities/Mental Retardation (DC-LD) (Royal College of Psychiatrists, 2001) represents a consensus of current professional opinion suggesting certain modifications that are appropriate for people with moderate to profound ID. The DC-LD allows both subjective description by the individual, or its observation by others as valid criteria for diagnosis.

The cognitive features of anxiety disorders are infrequently elicited from people with ID, while behavioural features are often seen. For example, restlessness and irritability are commonly observed in people with ID as symptoms of anxiety, and these can be quite severe. These symptoms have been included in the DC-LD criteria. Irritability may present as aggression towards self or others, or even destructiveness to property, and this can be a prominent part of clinical presentation of anxiety disorders, especially in those who are unable to describe their worries and fears.

As a result, the DC-LD excludes features such as depersonalisation and derealisation, which are complex cognitive phenomena, and for the diagnosis of phobias it does not require a recognition of the unreasonable nature of the fears as it was felt that people with ID may not have the requisite insight to recognise them as irrational. The emphasis is therefore on behavioural manifestations, such as restlessness and irritability, which in turn may manifest as aggression, self-injury or destructive behaviours.

As described previously, social withdrawal due to pervasive developmental disorders may indicate agoraphobia and social phobia, and these must be clearly differentiated. The diagnostic criteria for OCD in the general population also includes a description of a very complex cognitive phenomenon that would be very difficult to elicit from people with ID due to their limitations in verbal and cognitive skills. It is important that compulsions must be distinguished from repetitive movements, most often rhythmic movements, frequently seen in people with severe and profound ID (stereotypes).

The DSM–IV-TR (American Psychiatric Association, 2000), meanwhile, also advocates the need to capture additional clinical information that goes beyond the diagnosis to assist the process of assessment. It also emphasises the importance of clinical judgement and flexibility in the use of diagnostic criteria. This multi-axial approach accommodates physical illness, mental illness and other developmental disorders that may have a bearing on anxiety, and considers the varying assessments that might be made of symptoms, for example, that social withdrawal in pervasive developmental disorder needs to be differentiated from agoraphobia, and obsessions in pervasive developmental disorder distinguished from those seen in OCD. The Diagnostic Manual – Intellectual Disability (DM-ID) (Fletcher *et al*, 2007) is a similar adaptation of the DSM-IV-TR, and it also emphasises the different approaches to eliciting the required information.

Assessment instruments

Assessment instruments have the advantage of standardising information across time, assessors and contexts. These may include broadband scales covering a wide range of psychopathology and co-morbidities, and which tend to be longer, with varying psychometric properties for individual subscales. They are generally not useful in monitoring treatment effects. Narrowband instruments, meanwhile, focus on specific psychopathology whose subtypes can be explored. They also make for better baseline monitoring but do not allow the assessment of commonly co-morbid conditions.

Assessment instruments have varied in the use of self or informant reports. The advantages of each approach when dealing with people with ID are outlined in table 2.1.

Table 2.1: Self and informant reports	
Self report	Informant report
Advantages	Advantages
Access to subjective states.	Detailed objective account.
Access to sensitive information.	Perspectives on functioning, timelines and life events.
Cements therapeutic process.	Description of observed behaviours.
Disadvantages	Disadvantages
Interview-related anxiety might affect results.	Cannot always access subjective account.
Depends on cognitive abilities.	Subject to diagnostic overshadowing and preconceived bias.
Persons with ID might misunderstand, underestimate or minimise symptoms.	Depends of informant's knowledge and awareness.
Difficulties establishing timelines and precipitants.	Reliant on informant's relationship to the client.
Subject to limitations of insight and response bias.	

The choice of assessment instruments therefore depends on who is seeking what from whom and when, for example, clinical evaluations as compared to research, and population screening compared to diagnostic and prognostic considerations. The use of standardised instruments for the assessment of anxiety disorders presents particular difficulties in persons with ID because most of these instruments have been validated in the general population. There are particular challenges in ascertaining validity in people with moderate to severe ID as most scales call for an estimate of frequency and pervasiveness of symptoms. In recent years this has led to both adaptations to existing instruments as well as the development of instruments designed specifically for use in the ID population.

A recent systematic review has provided an overview of existing instruments for anxiety (Hermans *et al*, 2011) for details and references. Table 2.2 summarises the instruments reviewed.

Table 2.2: Overview of existing instruments

Name	Description	Advantages	Disadvantages
Glasgow Anxiety Scale (Mindham & Espie, 2003)	Screening. Narrow focus. Self-report. 24 items, three point ratings.	Validated in persons with ID. Robust psychometrics. Quick administration.	Needs further research into study of its psychometric properties.
Psychopathology Instrument for Mentally Retarded Adults – Self Report (PIMRA-SR) (Senatore et al, 1985)	Screening. Self-report. Broadband with seven item anxiety subscale. Based on DSM-III.	Assessment of co-morbid disorders.	Low to moderate reliability.
Zung Anxiety Rating Scale (Zung, 1971) adapted for persons with ID (Lindsay et al, 1994)	Self-report. Screening. 20 items.	Established provenance of the parent scale from which it is derived.	Low to moderate co-relations with other anxiety measures.
Fear Survey for Adults with Mental Retardation (FSAMR) (Ramirez & Lukenbill, 2007)	Screening. Self-report. 73 items.	Built–in acquiescence scale. Designed for persons with ID. Excellent internal consistency.	Poor correlation with other instruments.
The Anxiety, Depression and Mood Scale (ADAMS) (Esbensen et al, 2003)	Screening. Informant report. Seven item anxiety subscale with a four point rating. DSM-IV based.	Designed for persons with mild to moderate ID. Good psychometric properties.	Poor inter-rater reliability.

continued >

Name	Description	Advantages	Disadvantages
Assessment of Dual Diagnosis (ADD) (Matson & Bamburg, 1998)	Informant report. Screening instrument. 13 item anxiety subscale. Based on DSM-IV.	Designed for persons with mild to moderate ID.	
The Psychiatric Assessment Schedule for Adults with Developmental Disability Checklist (the PASS-AD) (Moss et al, 1998)	Screening. Broadband. Both informant and self-report. 29 items, four point rating.	Life events checklist. Good psychometric properties. Most robust of diagnostic instruments.	Anxiety state particularly difficult to diagnose (Costello et al, 1997).
The Mini Psychiatric Assessment Schedule for Adults with Developmental Disability Checklist (the Mini- PASS-AD) (Prosser et al, 1998)	Informant report. 84 items, four point rating. Anxiety and Phobia subscale.		Low to moderate psychometric properties.
The Diagnostic Assessment for the Severely Handicapped-II (DASH-II) (Matson, 1995)	Informant report. Broadband scale. Eight item anxiety subscale with a three point rating.	For persons with severe to profound ID.	Poor psychometrics but good inter-rater reliability.
The Psychopathology Instrument for Mentally Retarded Adults Informant (PIMRA-I) (Kazdin et al, 1983)	Informant rated. Broadband instrument. Anxiety disorder subscale.	Good test/re-test reliability.	

continued >

Name	Description	Advantages	Disadvantages
The Psychopathology in Autism Checklist (PAC) (Helverschou *et al*, 2009)	Informant rated. Six item anxiety subscale. Based in ICD 10 and DSM IV.	For persons with ID and autism.	Moderate reliability. Poor differentiation between different psychiatric diagnoses.
The Mood and Anxiety Semi-Structured Interview (MASS) (Charlot *et al*, 2007)	Diagnostic instrument Informant report. Based on DSM-IV-TR. 30-60 min interview.	Good validity. Can be administered by mental health professionals after minimal training.	
The Psychopathology Checklist for Adults with Intellectual Disability (P-AID) (Hove & Havik, 2008)	Diagnostic instrument. Informant rated. Five checklists for different anxiety disorders. Based on DC-LD.	Good psychometrics.	

Hermans *et al* (2011) are of the opinion that the GAS-AD was the most promising self-report instrument, the ADAMS the most promising informant-based instrument, and the PAS-ADD the most robust diagnostic instrument. However, the systematic review also highlighted that, for most instruments, the psychometric properties were insufficiently studied and there is a need for further research into the most promising existing instruments rather than the development of new instruments.

Case study: Mr X

Mr X was initially brought to the attention of the intensive support service for People with Learning Disabilities in 2009 at the age of 50. He has a mild learning disability (with an IQ of 56) and was experiencing new onset paranoid delusions and auditory hallucinations precipitated by the death of his long-term care giver. He was given a diagnosis of having a major depressive episode with psychotic features and was admitted to the inpatient assessment and treatment unit three times over the next eight months. On each occasion he was discharged back to his own home where he now lived alone.

Even when free of overt depressive symptoms, he occasionally called 999 for emergency medical service with complaints such as, *'I feel bad ... my chest hurts ... I feel like I am going to have a heart attack'*. The ambulance personnel would routinely transport him to the local emergency department where he was given benzodiazepines and then discharged to his GP.

Over the last two years, Mr X developed frequent somatic complaints, including chest pain, shortness of breath and stomach discomfort and fear. At times he would not leave his home for hours or days. He called the ambulance more frequently, and at times he threatened to commit suicide if he was not brought to A&E. He persistently said things such as, *'I feel bad ... I want to go to the hospital or I'll kill myself'*. However, he never harmed himself. He was then seen and assessed by the consultant psychiatrist for people with ID at the A&E department, where he denied being in a depressive mood.

It was also revealed that Mr X had made 52 calls to 999 in one year and in all instances the A&E doctors could not find any medical condition, but made note of a diagnosis of ID. The intensive support service then began to see Mr X, usually prompted by requests from the A&E department after a series of 999 calls.

continued >

During this period, a Mini PAS-ADD and questionnaire on panic symptoms that was adapted from the structured clinical interview for DSM-IV-TR was published. This questionnaire was given to Mr X about four times, who was seen in consultation three times for suicidal ideation and once for somatic symptoms. The ratings on the initial two questionnaires were inconsistent, and he was unable to complete the third one due to anxiety. However, his answers on the fourth questionnaire suggested that he had experienced nine of the 13 symptoms associated with a diagnosis of panic disorder as defined by DSM-III-R.

Three months later he was seen by a psychiatrist within the intensive support service where he was given 5mg of diazepam twice a day (a benzodiazepine). The intensive support service consultant psychiatrist who had been seeing him since also then added an antidepressant, fluoxetine, which produced a marked decrease in his symptoms of anxiety and panic. The records show that Mr X had fewer contacts with the A&E services after this time. Mr X now is able to visit his family and friends, go to the shop and perform his normal daily activities without calls to the ambulance service and costly and expensive visits through the ambulance and A&E system.

Mr X's presentation was unusual because his complaints lacked specificity. Given his level of cognitive functioning, he was unable to communicate effectively the level of anxiety associated with somatic symptoms. Initially, the A&E physicians did not pick up or understand his chief symptoms as being secondary to fear that panic attacks can produce. The panic disorder was initially not considered until it was screened through a structured questionnaire. In retrospect, panic attacks may have precipitated Mr X's calls to ambulance services, his visits to A&E department, his fears about returning home and possibly even his suicidal thoughts.

Accurate diagnosis of psychiatric disorders among people with ID will result in more effective treatment, possibly with fewer adverse effects. In the case of Mr X, antipsychotic medications had been prescribed. Once panic was considered, his condition responded much better to therapy with a selective serotonin reuptake inhibitor and a benzodiazepine.

Conclusion

Anxiety disorders are increasingly recognised as a common source of distress among people with ID. The recognition of anxiety disorder in this population entails a flexible approach that responds to their communication and cognitive styles, a knowledge of varied presentations across a range of abilities, and an understanding of the constitutional and environmental factors that may impact on the presentation.

It is also evident that these disorders are often under-diagnosed and untreated. The particular challenges to accurate recognition include the lack of available valid diagnostic systems and the mediating effects of developmental disabilities. It is hoped that diagnostic systems specifically adapted to persons with ID will mitigate some of these difficulties.

Summary

- Anxiety disorders are a common and treatable cause of distress and a change in functioning for people with ID.
- It is important to have flexible assessment approaches that accommodate varying cognitive abilities and styles, and to be aware of the varied risk factors in this population.
- Appropriate adaptations to diagnostic criteria and instruments should be used to maximise the validity of responses.

References

American Psychiatric Association (2000) *Diagnostic and Statistical Manual of Mental Disorders (4th edition).* Washington, DC: APA.

Bailey N & Andrews T (2003) Diagnostic criteria for psychiatric disorders for use with adults with learning disabilities/mental retardation (DC–LD) and the diagnosis of anxiety disorders. *Journal of Intellectual Disability Research* **47** (supplement 1) 50–61.

Bernstein G & Borchardt C (1991) Anxiety disorders in childhood and adolescence: A critical review. *Journal of the American Academy of Child and Adolescent Psychiatry* **30** (5) 19–532.

Borthwick-Duffy S & Eynman R (1990) Who are the dually diagnosed? *American Journal on Mental Retardation* **94** (6) 586–595.

Bourgeois J, Seritan A, Casillas E, Hessl D, Schneider A, Yang Y, Kaur I, Cogswell J, Nguyen D & Hagerman R (2011) Lifetime prevalence of mood and anxiety disorders in fragile X premutation carriers. *Journal of Clinical Psychiatry* **72** (2) 175–182.

Bregman J, Leckman J & Ort S (1988) Fragile X syndrome: genetic predisposition to psychopathology. *Journal of Autism Developmental Disorders* **18** (3) 343–354.

Budd E, Sigelman C & Sigelman L (1981) Exploring the outer limits of response bias. *Sociological Focus* **14** (4) 297–307.

Clarke D, Boer H, Whittington J, Holland A, Butler J & Webb T (2002) Prader-Willi syndrome, compulsive and ritualistic behaviours: the first population based survey. *British Journal of Psychiatry* **180** 358–362.

Charlot L, Deutsch C, Hunt A, Fletcher K & McLivane W (2007) Validation of the mood and anxiety semi-structured (MASS) interview for patients with intellectual disabilities. *Journal of Intellectual Disability Research* **51** (10) 821–834.

Cooper S (1997) Epidemiology of psychiatric disorders in elderly compared with younger adults with learning disabilities. *British Journal of Psychiatry* **170** 375–380.

Cooper S, Smiley E, Morrison J, Williams A & Allan L (2007) Mental ill health in adults with intellectual disabilities: prevalence and associated features. *The British Journal of Psychiatry* **190** 27–35.

Coplan D & Lydiard R (1998) Brain circuits in panic disorder. *Biological Psychiatry* **44** (12) 1264–1276.

Costello H, Moss S, Prosser H & Hatton C (1997) Reliability of the ICD 10 version of the Psychiatric Assessment Schedule for Adults with Developmental Disability (PAS-ADD). *Social Psychiatry and Psychiatric Epidemiology* **32** (6) 339–343.

Deb S & Iyer A (2004) Clinical interviews. In: P Sturmey (Ed) *Mood Disorders in People with Mental Retardation*. Kingston, NY: NADD Press.

Deb S, Thomas M & Bright C (2001) Mental disorder in adults with intellectual disability 1: prevalence of functional psychiatric illness among a community based population aged between 16 and 64 years. *Journal of Intellectual Disability Research* **45** (6) 495–505.

Dekker M & Koot H (2003) DSM-IV disorders in children with borderline to moderate intellectual disability, I: prevalence and impact. *Journal of the American Academy of Child and Adolescent Psychiatry* **42** (8) 915–922.

Duff R, La Rocca J, Lizzet A, Martin P, Pearce L, Williams M & Peck C (1981) A comparison of the fears of mildly retarded adults with children of their mental age and chronological age matched controls. *Journal of Behavioural Therapy and Experimental Psychology* **12** (2) 121–124.

Dykens E (2003) Anxiety, fears and phobias in persons with Williams syndrome. *Developmental Neuropsychology* **23** (1 & 2) 291–316.

Dykens E, Leckman J & Cassidy S (1996) Obsessions and compulsions in Prader-Willi syndrome. *Journal of Child Psychology and Psychiatry* **37** (8) 995–1002.

Edgerton R (1967) *The Cloak of Competence: Stigma in the lives of the mentally retarded*. Berkley, CA: University of California Press.

Edgerton R, Bollinger M & Herr B (1984) The cloak of competence: after two decades. *American Journal of Mental Deficiency* **88** (4) 345–351.

Emerson E (2003) Prevalence of psychiatric disorders in children and adolescents with and without intellectual disability. *Journal of Intellectual Disability Research* **47** (1) 51–58.

Esbensen A, Rojhan J, Aman M & Ruedrich S (2003) The reliability and validity of an assessment instrument for anxiety, depression and mood among individuals with mental retardation. *Journal of Autism and Developmental Disorders* **33** (6) 617–629.

Finlay W & Lyons E (2002) Acquiescence in interviews with people who have mental retardation. *Mental Retardation* **40** (1) 14–29.

Fletcher R, Loschen E, Stavrakaki C & First M (Eds) (2007) *NADD Diagnostic Manual – Intellectual Disability (DM-ID)*. Kingston, NY: NADD Press.

Gillott A & Standen P (2007) Levels of anxiety and sources of stress in adults with autism. *Journal of Intellectual Disabilities* **11**(4) 358–370.

Hagerman R (1996) Physical and behavioural phenotype. In: R Hagerman and A Cronister (Eds) *Fragile X Syndrome: Diagnosis, treatment, and research (2nd edition)* (pp3–87). Baltimore, MD: The John Hopkins University Press.

Heal L & Sigelman C (1995) Response bias in interviews of individuals with limited mental abilities. *Journal of Intellectual Disability Research* **39** (4) 331–340.

Helverschou S, Bakken T & Martinsen H (2009) The psychopathology in autism checklist (PAC): A pilot study. *Research in Autism Spectrum Disorders* **3** 179–175.

Hermans H, Van der Pas F & Evenhuis H (2011) Instruments assessing anxiety in adults with intellectual disabilities: a systematic review. *Research in Developmental Disabilities* **32** (3) 861-870.

Hove O & Havik O (2008) Psychometric properties of Psychopathology checklists for adults with intellectual disability (P-AID) on a community sample of adults with intellectual disability. *Research in Developmental Disabilities* **29** (5) 467–482.

Kashani J & Orvaschel H (1990) A community study of anxiety in children and adolescents. *American Journal of Psychiatry* **147** (3) 313–318.

Kazdin A, Matson J & Senaforce V (1983) Assessment of depression in mentally retarded adults. *American Journal of Psychiatry* **140** (8) 1040–1043.

Kessler R, McGonagle K, Zhao S, Nelson C, Hughes M, Eshleman S, Wittchen H & Kendler K (1994) Lifetime and 12-month prevalence of DSM-III-R psychiatric disorders in the United States: results from the National Co-morbidity Survey. *Archives of General Psychiatry* **51** (1) 716–722.

Khreim I & Mikkelson E (1997) Anxiety disorders in adults with mental retardation. *Psychiatric Annals* **27** (3) 271–281.

Lesch KP, Bengel D, Heils A, Sabol S, Greenberg B, Petri S, Benjamin J, Müller C, Hamer D & Murphy D (1996) Association of anxiety-related traits with a polymorphism in the serotonin transporter gene regulatory region. *Science* **274** (5292) 1527–1531

Lindsay W, Michie A, Baty F, Smith A & Miller S (1994) The consistency of reports about feelings and emotions from people with intellectual disability. *Journal of Intellectual Disability Research* **38** (1) 61–66.

Lund J (1988) Psychiatric aspects of Down's syndrome. *Acta Psychiatrica Scandinavica* **78** (3) 369–74.

Masi G, Brovedani P, Mucci M & Favilla L (2002) Assessment of anxiety and depression in adolescents with mental retardation. *Child Psychiatry and Human Development* **32** (3) 227–237.

Matson J (1995) *Diagnostic Assessment for the Severely Handicapped-II*. Baton Rouge: Scientific Publishers.

Matson J & Bamburg J (1998) Reliability of the assessment of dual diagnosis (ADD). *Research in Developmental Disabilities* **19** (1) 89–85.

Matson J, Smiroldo B, Hamilton M & Baglio C (1997) Do anxiety disorders exist in persons with severe and profound mental retardation? *Research in Developmental Disabilities* **18** (1) 39–41.

McEwen B (1998) Protective and damaging effects of stress mediators. *New England Journal of Medicine* **338** (3) 171–179.

Merikangas K & Kalaydjian A (2009) Epidemiology of anxiety disorders. In: B Sadock, V Sadock and P Ruiz (Eds) *Comprehensive Textbook of Psychiatry (9th edition)* (pp1856–1864). Philadelphia: Lippincot Williams and Wilkins.

Mikkelsen E & McKenna L (1999) Psychopharmacologic algorithms for adults with developmental disabilities and difficult-to-diagnose behavioural disorders. *Psychiatric Annals* **29** (5) 302–314.

Mindham J & Espie C (2003) Glasgow Anxiety Scale for people with an intellectual disability (GAS-ID): development and psychometric properties of a new measure for use with mild intellectual disability. *Journal of Intellectual Disability Research* **47** (1) 22–30.

Moss S (1999) Assessment: conceptual issues. In: N Bouras (Ed) *Psychiatric and Behavioural Disorders in Developmental Disabilities* (pp18-37). Cambridge: Cambridge University Press.

Moss S, Prosser H, Costello H, Simpson N, Patel P & Rowe S (1998) Reliability and validity of the PAS-ADD checklist for detecting psychiatric disorders in adults with intellectual disability. *Journal of Intellectual Disability Research* **42** (2) 173–183.

Myers B & Pueschel S (1991) Psychiatric disorders in a population with Down's syndrome. *Journal of Nervous and Mental Disease* **179** 609–13.

National Centre for Social Research (1997) *The National Psychiatric Morbidity Survey.* Leicester: University of Leicester.

Nelles W & Barlow D (1988) Do children panic? *Clinical Psychology Review* **8** (4) 889–909.

Nyhan W (1972) Behaviour phenotype in organic disease: presidential address to the Society of Pediatric Research, May 1, 1971. *Pediatric Research* **6** (1) 1–9.

Pickersgill M, Valentine J, May R & Brewin C (1994) Fears in Mental retardation: part one – types of fears reported by men and women with or without mental retardation. *Advances in Behavioural Research Therapy* **16** (4) 277–296.

Pine D (2009) Anxiety disorder: introduction and overview. In: B Sadock, V Sadock and P Ruiz (Eds) *Comprehensive Textbook of Psychiatry (9th edition)* (pp1839–1844). Philadelphia: Lippincot Williams and Wilkins.

Prosser H & Bromley J (1998) Interviewing people with intellectual disabilities. In: E Emerson, Hatton C and Bromley J (Eds) *Clinical Psychology and People with Intellectual disabilities* (pp99–113). London: John Wiley and Sons Ltd.

Prosser H, Moss S, Costello H, Simpson N, Patel P & Rowe S (1998) Reliability and validity of the Mini PAS-ADD for assessing psychiatric disorders in adults with intellectual disability. *Journal of Intellectual Disability Research* **42** (4) 264–272.

Raghavan R (1997) Anxiety disorders in people with learning disabilities: a review of the literature. *Journal of Learning Disabilities for Nursing, Health and Social Care* **2** (1) 3–9.

Ramierez S & Lukenbill J (2007) Development of the fear survey for adults with mental retardation. *Research in Developmental Disabilities* **28** (3) 225–237.

Rapley M (1995) Black swans: conversation analysis of interviews with people with learning disabilities. *Clinical Psychology Forum* **84** 17–23.

Reiss S, Levitan G & Szyszko J (1982) Emotional disturbance and mental retardation: diagnostic overshadowing. *American Journal of Mental Deficiency* **86** (6) 567–574.

Royal College of Psychiatrists (2001) *Diagnostic Criteria for Psychiatric Disorders For Use With Adults With Learning Disabilities / Mental Retardation (DC-LD): Occasional paper OP 48.* London: Gaskell.

Senatore V, Matson J & Kazdin A (1985) An inventory to assess psychopathology of mentally retarded adults. *American Journal of Mental Deficiency* **89** (5) 459–466.

Sigelman C, Budd E, Spanhel C & Shoenrock C (1981) Asking questions of retarded persons: A comparison of yes/no and either/or formats. *Applied Research in Mental Retardation* **2** (4) 374–57.

Silverman W & Nelles W (1990) Simple phobia in childhood. In: M Hersen and C Last (Eds) *Handbook of Child and Adult Psychopathology: A longitudinal perspective* (pp183–196). New York: Pergammon Press.

Skuse D (2000) Behaviour phenotypes: what do they teach us? *Archives of Diseases in Childhood* **82** (3) 222–225.

Sovner R (1986) Limiting factors in the use of DSM–III criteria with mentally ill/mentally retarded persons. *Psychopharmacology Bulletin* **22** (4) 1055–1059.

Stavrakaki C (2002) The DSM IV and how it applies to persons with developmental disabilities. In: D Griffiths, C Stavrakaki and J Summers (Eds) *Dual Diagnosis: An introduction to the mental health needs of persons with developmental disabilities* (pp115–149). Ontario: Habilitative Mental Health Resource Network.

Szymanski L, King B, Goldberg B, Reid A, Tonge B & Cain N (1998) Diagnosis of mental disorders in people with mental retardation. In: S Reiss and M Aman (Eds) *Psychotropic and Developmental Disabilities: The international consensus handbook* (pp3–17). Columbus, OH: Ohio State University, Nisonger Center.

Verhoeven W & Tuinier S (1997) Neuropsychiatric consultation in mentally retarded patients. *European Psychiatry* **12** (5) 242–248.

Wehmeyer M (1994) Reliability and acquiescence in the measurement of locus of control with adolescents and adults with mental retardation. *Psychological Reports* **75** (1 Pt 2) 527–537.

Wolff P, Gardner J, Paccla J & Lappen J (1989) The greeting behaviour of fragile X males. *American Journal of Mental Retardation* **93** (4) 406–411.

WHO (2010) *International Classification of Disorders.* Geneva: World Health Organisation.

Yerkes R & Dodson J (1908) The relation of strength of stimulus to rapidity of habit formation. *Journal of Comparative Neurology and Psychology* **18** (5) 459–482.

Zung W (1971) A rating instrument for anxiety disorders. *Psychosomatics* **12** (6) 371–379.

Chapter 3

Depressive disorders in people with intellectual disabilities

Tonye Sikabofori and Anupama Iyer

Overview

This chapter presents an overview of the presentation and manifestation of depressive disorders in people with ID. It explores the challenges facing practitioners in diagnosing and assessing depressive disorder across the range of cognitive abilities, and reviews risk factors for people with ID.

Learning objectives

- To understand the phenomenology of depressive disorders.
- To understand the presentation of depressive disorders in people with ID.
- To understand the various classification categories and the determinants and risk factors in people with ID.
- To review the assessment instruments for depressive disorders in people with ID.

Introduction

The occurrence of depressive disorders in persons with ID was described as early as the 19th century, and Wilber (1877) described melancholia and mania separate from mental retardation. Hurd (1888), meanwhile, described a range of depressive phenomenon including suicidal behaviours in persons with ID, and ID was acknowledged as a possible risk factor for the development of depression by Clouston (1883).

However, there were continuing conceptual doubts concerning the occurrence of syndromal affective disorders, especially in persons with severe ID (Earl, 1961; Sovner & Hurley, 1983). The 1980s saw a resurgence of interest in affective disorders in people with ID, when Reiss *et al* (1982) identified untreated emotional disorders as a significant unmet need in this population and Sovner and Hurley (1983) reviewed the existing studies and concluded that persons with ID experience the full range of affective disorders.

It has become increasingly acknowledged that depressive disorders significantly impair functioning and compromise community living (Jacobson & Schwartz, 1983). They also have a significant impact on families and carers (Bryne & Cunningham, 1985) and in increased costs of care.

Nature of depression

The basic affects, or emotions, such as joy, sadness, anger and fear, serve a communicative function and are expressed through facial expressions, vocal inflections, gestures and posture. Importantly, they tend to be short-lived in contrast to moods, which has been defined by the American Psychiatric Association as *'a pervasive and sustained emotion that, in the extreme, markedly colours one's perception of the world'* (APA, 2000). They are of a more enduring nature, conveying sustained emotions experienced long enough to be felt inwardly.

The normal everyday emotions of sadness should be differentiated from major depressive disorder. Sadness is a universal human response to defeat, disappointment or other adversities, and it may be adaptive in attempting to elicit support from significant others. Transient depressive periods also occur as reactions to specific stressors and loss. The expression of mood and affect may also be mediated by a person's affective temperament, which are inherent patterns or traits that develop in early life and determine a person's responses to events. These tend to vary in a relatively minor fashion in response and do not interfere with functioning. Temperaments tend to cluster into basic types and the depressive temperament, in which the person easily swings in the direction of sadness, occurs in three to six per cent of the general population.

Mood disorders, on the other hand, are characterised by predominant and persistent disturbances in mood, and they cover a variety of conditions of varying severity. These mood disturbances in turn lead to changes in cognitive appraisal of the self, the other and the future. They are also accompanied by changes in behaviours and biological functions, such as sleep, appetite and psychomotor functions. Mood disorders represent abnormal or extreme variations of mood that is out of proportion to any concurrent situation, or they arise without apparent life stress, are sustained for weeks or months, and have a pervasive effect on the person's judgement and functioning.

The ICD-10 (WHO, 2010) and the DSM-IV (APA, 2000) both categorise mood disorders into bipolar disorders (with manic or hypomanic, depressive, or mixed episodes) and major depressive disorders and their respective attenuated variants known as cyclothymic and dysthymic disorders.

Clinical features of depressive disorders in persons with ID

The symptoms of depression are many and varied, and they include:

- early morning waking
- sleeping too much
- losing or gaining weight
- loss of appetite
- low mood with or without diurnal variation
- anxiety
- social withdrawal
- loss of sexual interest
- loss of confidence
- self-blame and inappropriate guilt
- inability to make decisions
- difficulty concentrating
- slowed down thinking
- loss of functional or self-care skills
- thoughts of death
- suicidal thoughts/actions or other self-harming behaviour

- depressive delusions
- aggression
- irritability.

Low mood: many people who have experienced severe forms of depression would express feeling overwhelmed by their black moods, while others suggest that depression is like having an intense physical pain. It is much more than just feeling a bit low.

Loss of interest: people with ID who are depressed lose their zest for life and for their favourite pastimes. Everything seems an enormous effort, with lack of energy and constant tiredness being quite frequent features. These symptoms are more difficult to identify in people with greater degrees of ID, but there is no reason to suppose that the subjective sense of fatigue and loss of interest are not felt too.

Lowered energy: a common symptom in depression is fatigue, which may lead to visits to the GP. There may be a tendency to complain of physical aches and pains, as people with ID may have under-diagnosed physical health problems, and it is therefore important that the GP excludes physical health causes for any lack of energy first. Carers and family may find their lack of enjoyment difficult to understand or be sympathetic about, particularly when there is no obvious cause for depression.

Other features of depression may include anxiety and repetitive behaviours, obsessional thoughts, cognitive features and somatic features. It is not uncommon to find that depression triggers or increases certain kinds of challenging behaviours.

When a depressed person cannot communicate their feelings, it is important to be able to describe and monitor any behaviours that may suggest underlying depression. In two studies of depressed adults with Down's syndrome, the commonest symptoms were sadness, loss of interest, social withdrawal, reduced energy and slowed activity. However, in this group there are many more symptoms that have been described (Cooper & Collacott, 1994).

A lowered mood varies little from day to day and is often unresponsive to circumstances, yet may show a characteristic diurnal variation as the day goes on. As with manic episodes, the clinical presentation shows marked individual variations, and atypical presentations are particularly common in adolescents and in adults with ID. In some cases, anxiety, distress and motor agitation may at certain times be more prominent than features such as irritability, excessive consumption of alcohol and histrionic behaviour, while an increase in pre-existing phobic or obsessional symptoms or hypochondriacal preoccupations may also mask the depression, and the mood change. For depressive episodes, a duration of at least two weeks is usually required for diagnosis, but shorter periods may be reasonable if symptoms are unusually severe and of rapid onset.

Some of the above symptoms may be marked, and may develop characteristic features that are widely regarded as having special clinical significance. The most typical examples of these physical symptoms are:

- loss of interest or pleasure in activities that are normally enjoyable
- lack of emotional reactivity to normally pleasurable surroundings and events
- waking in the morning two or more hours before the usual time
- being particularly depressed in the morning
- objective evidence of definite psychomotor retardation or agitation (remarked on or reported by other people)
- marked loss of appetite
- weight loss (often defined as 5% or more of body weight in the past month)
- marked loss of libido.

In very severe depression, delusions, hallucinations or depressive stupor may sometimes be present. The delusions usually involve ideas of sin, poverty or imminent disasters, responsibility for which may be assumed by the patient. Auditory hallucinations are usually of defamatory or accusatory voices, while olfactory hallucinations are often of rotting filth or decomposing flesh.

Marston *et al* (1997) identified core features of depression, as described by diagnostic criteria, that were present in those with mild ID but, with increasing cognitive disabilities, only depressed mood and sleep disturbances retained their significance whereas screaming, self-injury and aggression were more frequently displayed. They described a checklist of symptoms commonly present in persons with ID that last two weeks or more:

- depressed effect
- tearfulness

- loss of interest
- lack of emotional response
- sleep disturbance (state type)
- diurnal variation of mood
- psychomotor agitation
- loss of appetite
- weight loss (5% body mass in one month)
- loss of libido
- loss of confidence
- unreasonable self-reproach
- suicidal ideation
- self-injurious behaviour
- delusion (mood congruents)
- loss of energy
- constipation
- anxiety
- obsessional/compulsive behaviour
- aggression
- irritability
- changeable mood
- reduced communication
- social liaison
- running away
- screaming
- anti-social behaviour
- stereotyped behaviour
- poor concentration.

Case study: Peter

Peter, a 20-year-old with severe ID and some autistic features, was causing himself serious injury. When he was first seen he had two black eyes from punching himself in the face, and lacerations on his chin from banging his head on the table.

He had a number of lacerations on the scalp stapled together as a result of constantly hitting his head. He was described by his carer as looking *'quite a pitiful sight'*. He could only be restrained with 24 hour, one-to-one nursing support. He would not say a word to the clinician who saw him, or even make eye contact. However, there was some other important information: while he was trying to hurt himself he was wailing miserably all the time, obviously greatly distressed. This was unusual as many self-injurious patients appear rather disassociated while hitting their heads or picking at their skin.

Further examination revealed that Peter was eating and sleeping poorly, and losing weight. The clinician was told that this behaviour began about six months earlier when his grandmother died. She was the only person to whom he related at all. He would run up to her when she visited him, while totally ignoring his parents.

A major depression was diagnosed, precipitated by bereavement. He was given antidepressants, which had a dramatic effect and his self-injurious behaviour stopped completely.

Epidemiology

Depression has been acknowledged as a major public health challenge with the World Health Organization (WHO) predicting that it will become the second leading contributor to the global burden of disease by 2020 (WHO, 2001). Ormel *et al* (2008) and Spijker *et al* (2004) suggested that depressive and anxiety disorders have a great impact on public health due to their negative effects on well-being, functioning and productivity. Both disorders often present a chronic intermittent cause, imposing a high disease burden throughout life. Most prognostic studies have found that basic clinical factors, such as early age of onset, severity and duration of the index episode, and co-morbidity of anxiety and depression, are among the most consistent and strong predictors (Spijker *et al*, 2004).

Since the 1980s, case reports have been replaced by large scale epidemiological studies of affective disorders in persons with ID. There has also been an attempt to delineate their presentation across the range of abilities. It is now acknowledged that depressed mood is among the most common of psychiatric symptoms experienced by adults with ID (Nezu *et al*, 1995). Major depression has, in fact, been reported in between one and five per cent of ID population (Cooper & Collacott, 1996; Lowry, 1998), and it may be that as many as one in 10 will experience clinical depression at some stage.

It is important to note that the risk of depression in persons with ID may be greater than that in the general population. Richards *et al* (2001) demonstrated that mild ID at the age of 15 was associated with a four-fold increase in affective disorders in midlife. It is also expected that, as in the general population, the risk of depression will increase with age (Thorpe, 1998).

An epidemiological investigation of affective disorders with a population based cohort study of 1,023 adults with ID was conducted by Cooper *et al* (2007). They found that the age-specific prevalence of depression as defined by the DC-LD was 4.9%. However, the point prevalence of depression, also defined by DC-LD, was:

- 3.8% for the group with mild ID
- 4.4% for the group with moderate ID
- 4.6% for the group with severe ID
- 2.2% for the group with profound ID.

The results show that the point prevalence was higher than previously reported for the general population, with DC-LD yielding 3.8% for depression and 0.6% for mania. Similar to the findings for the general population, depression was more associated with women and smoking, and rates were affected by preceding life events and the number of preceding family physician appointments. However, unlike the findings in the general population, obesity and unemployment were not independently associated with depression, nor was sensory impairment or a previous long stay in hospital residence. They therefore concluded that there is a high point prevalence of affective disorders in adults with ID.

Aetiology and risk factors of depressive disorders

A variety of genetic, biochemical, physical and psychosocial factors have been linked to affective disorders in the general population. However, people with ID are particularly vulnerable in some of these areas and for this reason they may be at increased risk of presenting with depressive features.

Biological factors

Many studies have reported biological abnormalities in people with mood disorders who have ID, and until recently the mono-immune neurotransmitters such as norepinephrine, dopamine, serotonin and histamine have been the main the focus of research as a possible cause. However, a progressive shift has now occurred towards studying neurobehavioural systems, neurocircuits and more intricate neuroregulatory systems.

Genetic factors

Numerous family, adoption and twin studies have long documented the heritability of mood disorders. Recently, however, the primary focus of genetic studies has been to identify specific genes that can make an individual susceptible by using molecular genetic methods. Feroz-Nainer (2005) made the point that epilepsy, FXS (see p30) and Down's syndrome are among the biological/genetic causes and correlates of ID, and he raised the question as to whether these factors also contribute to the higher rates of depression in people with mild ID.

Given the high prevalence of brain damage in the ID population, particularly in more severe ID, it is surprising that the role of organic factors such as epilepsy in the causation of depression has not been the subject of major reviews.

In his annual review of mental retardation, Rutter (1971) noted that children with ID accompanied by neurological abnormalities were more likely to have psychiatric diagnoses than those without such abnormalities. Lund (1985), meanwhile, in a study of 300 persons with ID, reported that

52% of people with both ID and epilepsy have a psychiatric diagnosis, compared to just 26% of those without epilepsy. Although this study did not examine a specific link with depressive disorder, Cornelius *et al* (1991) looked at the features of organic mood syndrome as presented by 130 patients with a variety of neurological disorders including epilepsy, cerebrovascular accidents and Parkinson's disease, and found a link between these organic syndromes and depression. Mendez *et al* (1994) further investigated the association between epilepsy and depression and found that the association may be particularly prominent with a left hemisphere lesion, especially those whose seizures originated from a structural brain lesion other than the mesial temporal sclerosis.

Psychosocial factors

It is a long-standing clinical observation that stressful life events more often precede the first episode of mood disorder than subsequent episodes. This association has been reported in both patients with major depressive disorder, and patients with bipolar disorder.

However, when it comes to ID, relatively few studies have examined the impact of life events on mental health, despite the possibility that people with ID might be particularly vulnerable to such events. McGillivray and McCabe (2007) maintained that disruptive life events, such as going into hospital, moving house, experiencing loss or separation from significant others, changes in family relationships or life-changing events, such as deaths in the family, are what can put persons with ID at risk of developing depression. Tsakanikos *et al* (2007) examined the impact of multiple life events on the mental health of people with ID and found that a single exposure to life events, both traumatic and non-traumatic, was significantly associated with schizophrenia, personality disorders and depression. Multiple exposures to life events were associated with personality disorder, depression and adjustment reaction, and these results suggest an increased vulnerability to life events in people with ID.

Day (1985), for example, explored the relationship between grief and depression in the psychoanalytic literature, and emphasised the difficulties facing people with ID in working through the grief process. Bereavement for an individual with ID may therefore be a particularly threatening life event resulting in a terrifying and rapid change in circumstances if someone close to them dies, especially if they were the individual's main carer (Harper & Wadsworth, 1993).

This view was also supported by Brown and Harris in their book, *The Social Origins of Depression* (1978), emphasising the importance of threatening life events in the genesis of depression, and the protective effects of intimate relationships and social support. People with ID often lack the skills to establish intimate relationships that could otherwise give some degree of protection, and they may be very isolated with poor systems of social support, particularly in community settings, thereby increasing their vulnerability to depression.

Personality factors

There is no single personality trait or type that uniquely predisposes a person to depression. All humans of whatever personality pattern can or do become depressed under certain circumstances. In the general population, however, people with certain personality disorders such as obsessive compulsive, histrionic and borderline, may be at greater risk of depression than people with antisocial or paranoid personality disorders.

John Bowlby (1973) believed that damaged early attachments and traumatic separation in childhood predispose the individual to depression. A loss that then occurs in adulthood will revive the memory of the traumatic childhood experience and so precipitate a depressive episode.

Lewinsohn (1974), meanwhile, proposed a model of depression that suggests that interactions between the individual and the environment lead to an increased vulnerability to depression. As many people with ID are relatively less competent in all areas than people in the normal IQ range, they experience negative reactions from family, peers, education and work settings, which may well lower self-esteem and lead to an increased vulnerability to depression.

Cognitive theory

According to cognitive theory, depression results from specific cognitive distortions that are present in people susceptible to depression, which are referred to as depressogenic schemata, and are a person's cognitive 'templates' that affect how they perceive both internal and external data, and which are altered by early experiences. Beck *et al* (1979) postulated a cognitive triad of depression that centres on a person's views of:

- the self ie. a negative self-perception
- the environment ie. a tendency to view the world as hostile and demanding
- the future ie. the expectation of suffering and failure.

In therapy, modifying these distortions is crucial.

Learned helplessness

The learned helplessness theory of depression connects depressive episodes to the experience of uncontrollable events where a person has both cognitive motivational deficit (they would not attempt to escape the event) and emotional deficit (indicating decreased reactivity to the event). This concept was introduced by Seligman (1981) who suggested that when an individual is faced with repeated failure they may begin to feel that they cannot change the situation for the better, and therefore assume a helpless response leading to a further deterioration in problem-solving behaviour and an increased vulnerability to depression. People with ID are particularly prone to failure because of basic deficits in understanding and problem-solving abilities, and are therefore more likely to assume a position of learned helplessness.

In their research on the early detection of depression and associated risk factors in adults with mild to moderate ID, McGillivray and McCabe (2007) described a number of cognitive factors that have been related to depression. They found, for example, links between depression and negative social comparison, poor self-concept and low self-esteem in this population. There is also evidence that severely depressed students with ID demonstrate a higher level of dysfunctional cognitive self-statements when compared to those who are not severely depressed, which suggests a need for further examination of the impact of cognitive factors on the development of depression in individuals with ID.

Diagnostic aspects

Recognising depressive disorders is not always easy, even in people without ID in primary care settings, with 50% of depressive illness being missed at first contact (Paykel & Priest, 1992), and this may well also be the true of persons with ID (Reynolds & Baker, 1988). In fact, recognising mental illness, including depression, in people with ID presents additional difficulties.

Not only might symptoms of an internalising non-disruptive nature not be recognised as a problem by carers (Marston *et al*, 1997), but the mediating effects of organic brain injury and additional genetic syndromes (Yappa & Roy, 1990) might further hamper recognition of an additional mental health concern. The reporting of symptoms may also be dependent upon the training and skills of care staff (Charlot *et al,* 1993), and may be confounded by the side effects of medication (Sovner & Hurley, 1983). In people with ID, depressive disorder may be difficult to diagnose because of impaired communication, and with this reduced ability to disclose their own moods, the psychiatrist is thereby denied access to the cardinal symptoms of affective illness (Einfeld, 1992). Furthermore, while people with mild ID may often be able to report their thoughts, feelings and emotions to another person, in the case of people with severe ID the psychiatrist must often rely on non-verbal cues from the client and behavioural observations from carers. In their report of five cases of bipolar illness in adolescents with a learning disability, McCraken and Diamond (1988) suggest that bipolar illness is commonly misdiagnosed in this population because of difficulties in eliciting histories of mood change and an overemphasis on psychotic and pseudo-organic symptoms. In many cases, symptoms such as reduced psychomotor activity, weight loss and sad facial expressions may be seen as non-disruptive, which lessens the likelihood that these clinical signs are regarded as a problem by carers.

Einfeld (1992) argues that mania tends to be over-diagnosed, as over-activity and excitement are common symptoms in this population. However, Charlot *et al* (1993) suggest that, as clinicians become more sensitive to the concern of the over diagnosis of mania, a downward trend in its occurrence might be expected.

Another major issue is the lack of diagnostic criteria for depression in people with ID. Standard general population diagnostic criteria such as ICD-10 or DSM-IV-TR are difficult to apply fully to people with severe and profound ID (see below). For example, a full understanding of complex concepts such as guilt and worthlessness require a developmental level of about seven years, and those without verbal communication skills would be unable to report recurrent thoughts of death, suicidal ideation or diminished ability to think, therefore limiting the usefulness of such items (Smiley & Cooper, 2003).

However, it is reported that the pragmatic application of standardised diagnostic criteria could, to an extent, overcome this problem. Indeed, studies by Meins (1995) and Marston *et al* (1997) suggest that standardised diagnostic criteria, such as DSM-IV and ICD-10, can be effectively used to detect depression associated with mild ID, but this criteria may be less useful for people with more severe disabilities.

Sovner and Hurley (1982) were the first to postulate that mood disorders may present atypically in persons with ID, and they proposed the term 'behavioural equivalents' to describe these alternative behavioural manifestations. Lowry and Sovner (1992) further delineated these 'symptomatic behaviours' based on a review of case notes as well as clinical experience. It was postulated that these observable behaviours would complement both self and informant reports. In this model, behavioural equivalents elaborated on symptoms of depression found in the non-disabled population but did not replace them.

Langlois and Martin (2008) looked at the relationship between diagnostic criteria, depressive equivalents and diagnosis of depression among older adults with ID. They looked at the criteria in the interRAI-ID assessment instrument that are representative of the DSM-IV criteria, and depressive equivalents were examined among persons with ID in an institution and in community based residential settings. They found that the DSM-IV diagnostic criteria and depressive equivalents were significantly related to a diagnosis of depression among older and younger adults with ID. The results show that a non-trivial proportion of persons in the study exhibited both DSM-IV criteria related to sad mood and somatic symptoms, and that the depressive equivalents were also common where aggression and self-injurious behaviour were the most prevalent. They also found that adults without a diagnosis of depression tended to exhibit self-injurious behaviour less frequently than younger adults, although rates for all other indicators were unaffected by age.

Tsiouris *et al* (2004) used the Bayesian analysis of the Clinical Behaviour Checklist for Persons with Intellectual Disabilities (CBCPID) (Marston *et al*, 1997) to predict depression in people with ID. This checklist was administered to 92 adults with ID who had been referred for psychiatric assessment, and compared the presence or absence of each criterion to the presence or absence of a diagnosis of depression by a psychiatrist. The study found only one item with adequate sensitivity (anxiety) and a few items with adequate specificity (suicidality, self-reproach, weight loss, constipation, loss of appetite, antisocial behaviour, loss of confidence, running away and psychomotor agitation). Although ideally the items should have both high sensitivity and specificity, unfortunately no items in this analysis had that property.

Adaptation to diagnostic systems

The use of structured interviews in conjunction with fully operationalised criteria has had a major impact on the overall reliability of the psychiatric diagnosis process.

There is, however, some debate about the use of such diagnostic tools when they are applied to people with ID. Some argue that the existing psychiatric nosological systems fall short when they are applied to this population, and several reviews over the last three decades (Cooper & Collacott, 1996; Davis *et al*, 1997; Janowsky & Davis, 2005) have found that the use of unmodified ICD-10 and DSM diagnostic systems is inappropriate, especially for those with severe ID. It has been stated, on the other hand, that standard diagnostic criteria may be appropriate for mild to moderate ID (Pawlarcyzk & Beckwith, 1987; Tsiouris, 2001; McBrien, 2003).

Authors have highlighted the risks of both false negatives due to under recognition (McBrien, 2003) and false positives with increased rates observed when using symptoms equivalents (Davis *et al*, 1997; Holden & Gitelsen, 2004). McBrien (2003) has presented a comprehensive review of the various historical alternatives and modifications to DSM and ICD criteria.

The National Association for the Dually Diagnosed, in collaboration with the APA, adapted the DSM-IV-TR for use with individuals with ID. It has been recognised that the Diagnostic Manual – Intellectual Disability (DM-ID) is easy to use, accurate and can reduce residual categories (Fletcher *et al*, 2009). It provides clear examples of how criteria should be interpreted when used on people with ID, addressing the pathoplastic effects of ID on psychopathology.

Following a review of current literature, it was agreed that DSM-IV-TR mood disorder criteria did not need to be changed in significant ways, and the effort should aim at improving reliability and validity in eliciting existing criteria for this population (Charlot *et al*, 2007). The report recommended that some symptoms should be given differential emphasis, for instance irritability may present frequently as sadness (Charlot, 1997; Davis *et al*, 1997). It also suggests stipulating four or more symptoms (instead of five) required by DSM-IV-TR.

The DM-ID emphasises the need for a '*change from what is usually observed for the individual*'. This can include an onset of, or an increase in, '*agitated behaviours*' (assaults, self-injury, disruptive or destructive behaviours) as well as stereotypes and ritualistic behaviours. It also provides guidance on the manner in which these symptoms may present to observers, for example weight loss may present as refusing meals, or exhibiting agitated behaviours at meal times such as throwing food and screaming when meals arrive. It has been suggested that psychomotor agitation may present more commonly in persons with ID, but Charlot *et al* (1997) has described a combination of withdrawn, underactive behaviours alternating with agitated, restless behaviours in response to demands. It also emphasises ruling out physical problems causing pain or distress such as infections, constipation or medication-induced side effects.

The DC-LD represents the consensus of current professional opinion and suggests modifications that are appropriate for people with moderate to profound ID and uses the hierarchical approach in order to place problem behaviours within the diagnostic framework with clear instructions regarding organic disorders and behavioural phenotypes. It also has items within categories that accommodate the pathoplastic effect of more severe ID and replaces some of the self-report items with observable items (Smiley & Cooper, 2003).

The DC-LD suggests eliminating the requirement for more cognitively based symptoms, such as excessive feelings of guilt and unworthiness, pessimistic views about the future and ideas of self-harm, and instead includes other symptoms such as an increase in specific maladaptive behaviours concurrent with episodes of mood disorder or the recent onset of, or increase in, physical health symptoms. Other examples include anhedonia (loss of ability to experience pleasure), which may manifest in an apparent loss of skills and non-compliance with care, and loss of confidence, which may manifest as an increase in fearfulness and reassurance seeking.

The DM-ID was also designed to consider the developmental perspective in order to aid the clinician in recognising symptom profiles in children with ID as well.

Assessment tools

Several scales are needed, both as screening tools to evaluate the need for further assessment, and to evaluate the trajectory of a particular episode. Some of the scales are derived from those designed for use with the general population, however more recently several instruments have been designed and validated specifically for people with ID.

As has already been discussed, there are various challenges to be faced when assessing depressive disorders in people with ID, and Reynolds and Baker (1988) highlighted the particular problems with using self-report questionnaires, which are reliant on both expressive and receptive language abilities. They also expressed their concerns regarding the lack of psychometric data available for scales modified for use with ID. Feinstein *et al* (1988), meanwhile, highlighted the mediating effects of immaturity in children and adolescents with ID.

Feinstein *et al* (1988) suggested that a scale should ideally be able to assess a broad range of different moods, and the emphasis should be on behavioural descriptions using verbal information as supplementary data. It also eschewed brief interview formats, instead encouraging extended informant observations in naturalised settings, including measuring both frequency and severity of depressive episodes.

Table 3.1 summarises some of the instruments used in the assessment of mood disorders in persons with ID.

Table 3.1: Summary of assessment instruments

Name	Description	Advantages	Disadvantages
The Mini PAS-ADD Interview (Prosser et al, 1998)	86 items. Covers a range of psychiatric disorders. Informant rated.	Complements psychiatric assessment but does not replace it as it does not provide a diagnosis.	Training required. Psychometric data is limited to the overall scale rather than affective subscale in particular, hence validity statistics is limited.
PAS-ADD checklist revised (Moss et al, 1998)	25 items covering a range of disorders. Informant rated. Screening and monitoring affective disorder items.	Can be used with severe ID. No training needed. Uses 'everyday' language.	Needs two raters. Some concerns about untrained raters to use the checklist.
Clinical Behaviour Checklist for Persons with Intellectual Disabilities (CBDPID) (Marston et al, 1997)	30 item symptom checklist. 5 item scale delivered by Tsouris et al (2003).	Based on ICD-10 symptoms for depression. Brief measure. Reasonable psychometric properties.	Needs psychiatric input. Further studies needed into its scope and utility.
Children's Depression Inventory (CDI) (Kovacs, 1985)	27 items based on Beck Depression Inventory. Both self and informant formats. All levels of ID.	Pictorial response scales. Probes to check understanding. Reasonable psychometric properties.	Depends on level of cognitive and linguistic abilities. Some doubts have been raised about informants rating complex internal states.

Table 3.1: Summary of assessment instruments (continued)

Glasgow Depression Scale for People with Learning Disability (GDS-LD) (Cuthill et al, 2003)	Self report. Screening Instrument. 20 items for use with mild to moderate ID.	Based on DC-LD criteria. Uses symbols anchoring events and alternative phasing. Informant version with good psychometric properties and good interaction correlations with self-rating scales.	New scale, more research needed reading the psychometric properties of the instrument.
Psychopathology Inventory for Mentally Retarded Adults (PIMRA) (Senatore et al, 1985)	56 item broadband scale. Screening tool. 7 item affective disorder. Section for persons with mild ID.	Not specific to depression. From DSM-III. Simplified descriptions. Psychometrics for individual scales are not as robust.	Adapted assessment to co-morbid disorders.

Case study

A 34-year-old man with moderate ID and FXS (based upon chromosomal analysis) presented with a one-year history of increasing aggression and loss of functioning. Three of his four brothers also had chromosomal evidence of FXS. The patient was in good health, living in a community residence, and had been in care between the ages of 11 and 31. As a child he had been treated with stimulant therapy for hyperactivity. He was admitted to a psychiatric hospital at the age of 32 to control his aggressive behaviour and treatment has predominantly used neuroleptics, which has been largely ineffective.

At the time of his initial assessment he was taking chlorpromazine (200mg), trifluoperazine (10mg x 2 per day) and benzatropine (2mg). His behavioural problems included agitation and aggressiveness and he was easily frustrated and distractible, while he also said unusual things such as claiming that he was his brother. He also had orofacial dyskinesia, which was observed as the trifluoperazine was tapered off.

A diagnosis of organic personality disorder was considered and over an 18-month period the chlorpromazine was slowly withdrawn. During this period his aggressive behaviour began to increase and beta blocker therapy was tried, but this proved unsuccessful and was stopped due to hypertension. His clinical status was reassessed and a diagnosis of depressive disorder was given. He was therefore treated with antidepressants, which proved effective after eight weeks as his features reduced to a manageable level, he was a lot happier and the activities in his daily life were improved.

Conclusion

Depressive disorders are increasingly recognised as among the most common source of distress for people with ID. Diagnosis in those with ID entails a flexible approach that responds to the communication and cognitive styles of the person, a sound knowledge of the varied presentations across a range of skills, and a good understanding of the constitutional and environmental factors that may impact on presentations.

The particular challenges to accurate recognition include the lack of availability of valid diagnostic systems and the mediating effects of the developmental disabilities. Hopefully, diagnostic systems specifically adapted to persons with ID will mitigate some of these difficulties.

Summary

- The risk of depression in persons with ID may be greater than that in the general population.

- Depressive disorders significantly impair functioning, compromise community living and lead to significant morbidity in the form of self-injury and other maladaptive behaviours. They also have a significant impact on families and carers and increased costs of care.

- The recognition of depressive disorders in persons with ID poses additional challenges.

- Diagnostic systems and assessment instruments specifically adapted to people with ID will improve the recognition of this potentially treatable condition.

References

APA (2000) *Diagnostic and Statistical Manual of Mental Disorders* (4th edition) (DSM–IV–TR). Washington, DC: American Psychiatric Association.

Beck A, Rush A, Shaw B & Emery G (1979) *Cognitive Therapy of Depression*. New York: Guilford Press.

Bowlby J (1973) *Attachment and Loss*. New York: Basic Books.

Brown G & Harris T (1978) *The Social Origins of Depression*. London: Tavistock Publications.

Bryne E & Cunningham C (1985) The effects of mentally handicapped children on families: a conceptual review. *Journal of Child Psychology and Psychiatry* **26** (6) 847–846.

Charlot L (1997) Irritability, aggression and depression in adults with mental retardation: a developmental perspective. *Psychiatric Annals* **27** 190–197.

Charlot L, Doucette A & Mezzacappa E (1993) Affective symptoms of institutionalised adults with mental retardation. *American Journal of Mental Retardation* **98** (3) 408–416.

Charlot L, Fox S, Silka V, Hurley A, Lowry M & Parry R (2007) Mood disorders. In: R Fletcher, E Loschen, C Stavrakaki and M First (Eds) *NADD Diagnostic Manual – Intellectual disability (DM-ID)*. Kingston, NY: NADD Press.

Clouston T (1883) *Clinical Lectures on Mental Diseases*. London.

Cooper S & Collacott R (1994) Clinical features and diagnostic criteria of depression in Down's syndrome. *British Journal of Psychiatry* **165** (3) 399–403.

Cooper S & Collacott R (1996) Depressive episodes in adults with intellectual disabilities. *Irish Journal of Psychological Medicine* **13** 105–113.

Cooper S, Smiley E, Morrison J, Williamson A & Allan L (2007) An epidemiological investigation of affective disorders with a population-based cohort of 1,023 adults with intellectual disabilities. *Psychological Medicine* **37** (6) 873–882.

Cornelius J, Mezzich J, Fabrega H, Cornelius M, Myers J & Ulrich R (1991) Characterizing organic hallucinosis. *Comprehensive Psychiatry* **32** (4) 338–344.

Cuthill F, Espie C & Cooper S (2003) Development and psychometric properties of the Glasgow Depression Scales for people with a learning disability: individual and carer supplement versions. *British Journal of Psychiatry* **182** 347–353.

Davis J, Judd F & Herman H (1997) Depression in adults with intellectual disability part 1: a review. *Australian and New Zealand Journal of Psychiatry* **31** (2) 232–242.

Day K (1985) Psychiatric disorders in the middle-aged and elderly mentally handicapped. *British Journal of Psychiatry* **147** 660–667.

Earl C (1961) *Subnormal Personalities*. London: Baillierre.

Einfeld S (1992) Clinical assessment of psychiatric symptoms in mentally retarded individuals. *Australian and New Zealand Journal of Psychiatry* **26** (1) 48–63.

Feinstein C, Kaminea Y, Barrett R & Tylenda B (1988) The assessment of mood of affect in developmentally disabled children and adolescents: the emotional disorders rating scale. *Research in Developmental Disabilities* **9** (2) 109–121.

Feroz-Nainer C (2005) Confounding factors for depression in adults with mild learning disability. *British Journal of Psychiatry* 187: 89 doi:10.1192.

Fletcher R, Havercamp S, Ruedrich S, Benson B, Barnhill L, Cooper S & Stavrakaki C (2009) Clinical usefulness of Diagnostic Manual Intellectual Disability (DM-ID) for mental disorders in persons with intellectual disability: results from a brief field Survey. *Journal of Clinical Psychiatry* **70** (7) 967–974.

Harper D & Wadsworth J (1993) Grief in adults with mental retardation: preliminary findings. *Research in Developmental Disabilities* **14** (4) 313–330.

Holden B & Gitelsen J (2004) The association between severity of intellectual disability and psychiatric symptomatology. *Journal of Intellectual Disability Research* **48** (6) 556–562.

Hurd H (1888) Imbecility and insanity. *Journal of Insanity* **45** 263–371.

Jacobson J & Schwartz A (1983) Personal and service characteristics affecting group home placement success: a prospective analysis. *Mental Retardation* **21** (1) 1–7.

Janowsky D & Davis J (2005) Diagnosis and treatment of depression in patients with mental retardation. *Current Psychiatry Reports* **7** (6) 421–428.

Kovacs M (1985) The Children's Depression Inventory (CDI). *Psychopharmacology Bulletin* **21** (4) 995–998.

Langlois L & Martin L (2008) Relationship between diagnostic criteria, depressive equivalents and diagnosis of depression among older adults with intellectual disability. *Journal of Intellectual Disability Research* **52** (11) 896–904.

Lewinsohn P (1974) A behavioural approach to depression. In: R Friedman and M Katz (Eds) *The Psychiatry of Depression: Contemporary theory and research* (pp157–185). New York: Wiley.

Lowry M & Sovner R (1992) Severe behaviour problems associated with rapid cycling bipolar disorder in two adults with profound mental retardation. *Journal of Intellectual Disabilities Research* **36** (3) 269–281.

Lowry M (1998) Assessment and treatment of mood disorders in persons with developmental disabilities. *Journal of Developmental and Physical Disabilities* **10** (4) 387–406.

Lund J (1985) Epilepsy and psychiatric disorder in the mentally retarded adult. *Acta Psychiatrica Scandinavica* **72** (6) 557–562.

Marston G, Perry D & Roy A (1997) Manifestations of depression in people with intellectual disability. *Journal of Intellectual Disability Research* **41** (6) 476–480.

McBrien J (2003) Assessment and diagnosis of depression in people with intellectual disability. *Journal of Intellectual Disability Research* **47** (1) 1–13.

McCracken J & Diamond R (1998) Bipolar disorder in mentally retarded adolescents. *Journal of the American Academy of Child and Adolescent Psychiatry* **27** 494–499

McGillivray J & McCabe M (2007) Early detection of depression and associated risk factors in adults with mild/moderate intellectual disability. *Research in Developmental Disabilities* **28** (1) 59–70.

Meins W (1995) Symptoms of major depression in mentally retarded adults. *Journal of Intellectual Disabilities Research* **39** (1) 41–45.

Mendez M, Taylor J, Doss R & Salguero P (1994) Depression in secondary epilepsy: relation to lesion laterally. *Journal of Neurology, Neurosurgery and Psychiatry* **57** (2) 232–233.

Merrick J, Merrick E, Lunsky Y & Kandel I (2005) Suicide behaviour in persons with intellectual disability. *Scientific World Journal* **5** 729–735.

Moss S, Prosser H, Costello H, Simpson N, Patel P, Rowe S, Turner S & Hatton C (1998) Reliability and validity of the PAS-ADD Checklist for detecting psychiatric disorders in adults with intellectual disability. *Journal of Intellectual Disability Research* **42** (2) 173–183.

Nezu C, Nezu A, Rothenberg J, Dellicaipini L & Groag I (1995) Depression in adults with mild mental retardation – are cognitive variables involved? *Cognitive Therapy and Research* **19** (2) 227–239.

Ormel J, Petukhova M, Chatterji S, Aguilar-Gaxiola S, Alonso J, Angermeyer M, Bromet E, Burger H, Demyttenaere K, de Girolamo G, Haro J, Hwang I, Karam E, Kawakami N, Lepine J, Medina-Mora M, Posada-Villa J, Sampson N, Scott K, Ustun T, von Korff M, Williams D, Zhang M & Kessler R (2008) Disability and treatment of specific mental and physical disorders across the world: results from the WHO world health surveys. *British Journal of Psychiatry* **192** (5) 368–375.

Pawlarcyzk D & Beckwith B (1987) Depressive symptoms displayed by persons with mental retardation: a review. *Mental Retardation* **25** (6) 323–30.

Paykel E & Priest R (1992) Recognition and management of depression in general practice: consensus statement. *The British Medical Journal* **305** (6863) 1198–1202.

Prosser H, Moss S, Costello H, Simpson N, Patel P & Rowe S (1998) Reliability and validity of the Mini PAS-ADD for assessing psychiatric disorders in adults with intellectual disability. *Journal of Intellectual Disability Research* **42** (4) 264–272.

Reiss S, Levitan G & Szyszko J (1982) Emotional disturbance and mental retardation: diagnostic overshadowing. *American Journal of Mental Deficiency* **86** (6) 567–574.

Reynolds W & Baker J (1988) Assessment of depression in persons with mental retardation. *American Journal on Mental Retardation* **93** (1) 93–103.

Richards M, Maughan B, Hardy R, Hall I, Strydom A & Wadsworth M (2001) Long term affective disorder in people with mild learning disability. *British Journal of Psychiatry* **179** 523–527.

Rutter M (1971) Psychiatry. In: J Wortis (Ed) *Mental Retardation and Developmental Disabilities: An annual review.* New York: Grure & Stratton.

Seligman E (1981) A learned helplessness point of view. In: L Rehm (Ed) *Behaviour Therapy for Depression: Present status and future directions* (pp123–42). New York: Academic Press.

Senatore V, Matson J & Kazdin A (1985) An inventory to assess psychopathology of mentally retarded adults. *American Journal of Mental Deficiency* **89** (5) 459–466.

Smiley E & Cooper S (2003) Intellectual disabilities, depressive episode and diagnostic criteria for psychiatric disorders for use with adults with learning disabilities/mental retardation (DC-LD). *Journal of Intellectual Disability Research* **47** (supplement 1) 62–71.

Sovner R & Hurley A (1982) Diagnosing depression in the mentally retarded. *Psychiatric Aspects of Mental Retardation Reviews* **1** 1–3.

Sovner R & Hurley A (1983) Do the mentally retarded suffer from affective illness? *Archives of General Psychiatry* **40** (1) 61–67.

Spijker J, De Gruaf R, Bigh R, Beekman A, Ormel J & Nolen W (2004) Determinants of persistence of major or depressive episodes in the general population. Results from the Netherlands Mental Health Survey and Incidence Study (NEMESIS). *Journal of Affective Disorders* **81** (3) 231–240.

Thorpe L (1998) Psychiatric Disorders. In: M Janicki and P Datton (Eds) *Dementia and Ageing Adults with Intellectual Disabilities: A handbook* (pp217–231). Philadelphia: Brunzer/Mazel.

Tsakanikos E, Bouras N, Costell H & Hott G (2007) Multiple exposure to life events and clinical psychopathology in adults with intellectual disability. *Social Psychiatry and Psychiatric Epidemiology* **42** (1) 24–28.

Tsiouris J (2001) Diagnosis of depression in people with severe/profound intellectual disability. *Journal of Intellectual Disability Research* **45** (2) 115–120.

Tsiouris J, Mann R, Patti P & Sturmey P (2004) Symptoms of depression and challenging behaviour in people with intellectual disability: A Bayesian analysis. *Journal of Intellectual and Developmental Disability* **29** (1) 65–69.

Wilbur H (1877) The classification of idiocy. In: *Proceedings of the Association of Medical Officers of American Institutions for Idiotic and Feeble-Minded persons* (pp29–35). Philadelphia: Lippincott.

WHO (2001) *The World Health Report 2001 Mental Health: New understanding, new hope.* Geneva: World Health Organisation.

WHO (2010) *International Classification of Disorders.* Geneva: WHO.

Yappa P & Roy A (1990) Depressive illness and mental handicap: two case reports. *Journal of the British Institute of Mental Handicap* **18** (1) 19–21.

Chapter 4

User views and experiences

Eddie Chaplin and Steve Hardy

Overview

This chapter examines the thoughts and opinions of people with ID on anxiety and depression. It offers insights into what they think makes people vulnerable to these mental health problems and what can protect them from developing them. Two individuals also offer personal insights into their experiences. The chapter includes a brief description of an organisational model that has been developed to ensure that the voices of people using services are heard in all areas of an organisation. It concludes by describing how the opinions of people with ID were used to develop a guided self-help tool called the Self-Assessment and Intervention (SAINT).

Learning objectives

- To begin to understand the issues that are important to service users with ID and mental health needs.
- To understand ways of developing meaningful service user involvement at different levels within organisations.
- To understand ways in which people with ID are able to participate in their care with or without support.

Introduction

The involvement of people with ID in all aspects of the support and services they receive has been steadily growing in momentum over the last 30 years. The inclusion agenda has been a consistent and central theme to government policy (Adults with Incapacity (Scotland) Act (2000); DH, 2001, 2009; DHSS, 2005; Welsh Office, 2001), and it is now not only common but expected practice that people with ID contribute to service development, evaluation, education and training, as well as being full partners in their own care.

However, for those with ID and additional mental health problems, often a marginalised group who had in the past fallen between the eligibility criteria of services, the inclusion agenda was somewhat slower. This was addressed at policy level in England and Wales in 2004 by the introduction of the Green Light Tool Kit (FPWLD, 2004), a self-assessment toolkit that included standards on involving service users. Other reports have specifically addressed the views and opinions of people with ID who have mental health problems (Cole, 2002; Estia Centre, 2003), who have reported similar accounts, such as problems accessing local services, a lack of trained staff and poor levels of support.

Regarding national mental health policy, *No Health Without Mental Health* (DH, 2011), lay out the government's strategy for improving outcomes for people with mental health problems in England. An underpinning theme was the involvement of those who use services:

'Put them and their families and carers at the centre of their care by listening to what they want, giving them information, involving them in planning and decision making, treating them with dignity and respect, and enabling them to have choice and control over their lives and the services they receive.' (DH, 2011, p16)

What do people with ID think about anxiety and depression?

For the purpose of this chapter, eight people with ID were interviewed, all of whom had used or were using mental health services. We wanted to explore what anxiety and depression meant to them, but also what might make them vulnerable to developing anxiety or depression, and what could help protect them.

Here are some of their responses.

What does anxiety mean to you?

- Anxiety is when you feel nervous.
- It's when you worry all the time.
- Sometimes it's so bad that someone can't leave the house.
- Some people have phobias, of spiders or dogs.
- You might get anxious when you have to move somewhere new.
- Anxiety can be terrible.

What does depression mean to you?

- Depression is when you feel sad all the time.
- You might get depressed when someone dies or a friend moves away.
- Depression can be very serious. It can stop you enjoying your life.

What things can make someone become anxious or depressed?

- Abuse.
- Being bored.
- Discrimination.
- Having no one to talk to.
- If people don't understand you.
- Not having enough money.
- Too much alcohol or using drugs.

What things that can help people stay well or get better?

- Feeling safe.
- Getting enough sleep.
- Having a boyfriend or girlfriend.
- Having a job or things to do in the daytime.
- Healthy eating and being a good weight.
- Keeping fit.
- Having a social life.

- Someone to share your problems with.
- Standing up for your rights.

What can people do if they are anxious or depressed?

- Talk to family, friends or staff.
- Do something you like to take your mind off it.
- Learn relaxation exercises or meditation.
- See a psychologist or counsellor.
- The doctor can give you medication.
- Do mood charts and have coping strategies.
- If it gets really bad, call the Samaritans or go to A & E.

Anxiety: a personal account

What does anxiety mean to you?
'Sometimes I get anxious and I worry a lot. I get frightened. I start to shake, my heart beats faster. I scratch myself when I am anxious. I need more support when I am anxious.'

What makes you feel anxious?
'I'm scared of heights. I don't like walking up hills or long stairs. Also crowded places make me have panic attacks.'

Can you give an example of when you felt anxious?
'I was going to talk at a conference in Camden. We got the tube from London Bridge, the platform was very busy. I thought I was going to fall onto the train track, I become very anxious. My heart was beating faster and faster and I had trouble breathing. I walked back from the platform so I could calm down. I waited for 10 minutes until I could get on a tube.'

What helps you with your anxiety?
'I see a psychologist who helps me with my anxiety. We talk about the things that make me anxious and how to cope. I practice deep breathing exercises and I have a stress ball. My key worker helps me plan what times I am going to use the bus or tube and the best time to go shopping.'

Anxiety and Depression in People with Intellectual Disabilities   © Pavilion Publishing and Media Ltd 2012

Depression: a personal account

Can you tell us about when you were depressed?

*'A few years back I had to stay in hospital. I had a mental health problem –
I had very bad depression. I wasn't looking after myself, my flat was really
messy. I stopped going to college. I wasn't eating properly. I was hearing
voices, they were saying horrible things. I was very frightened. I needed help.'*

What help did you get?

*'I went to stay in a ward for people with mental health problems. It was for
people with learning disabilities. I agreed to stay there until I got better.*

*On the ward I had a psychiatrist and my own nurse. I had my own room.
They gave me medication for the depression; it helped a lot. The occupational
therapist helped me be independent again. I went to lots of groups, like a
relaxation group, a community group and the gym. The staff were friendly
and helpful. I always had someone to talk to.*

*I still saw my community psychiatric nurse when I was on the ward and
my support workers as well. They helped plan what would happen when I
went home.'*

Getting heard

In mental health services, people's experiences often go unheard. In the
South London and Maudsley NHS Foundation Trust there is a growing
service user movement helping to shape services. As well as producing
feedback questionnaires to inform performance, it also gives those using
services a voice across organisational forums.

One of the trust's services, the Behavioural and Developmental Psychiatry
Clinical Academic Group (CAG), has developed a two-tier approach to ensure
user and carer involvement and to make sure that users' views are heard
across all tiers of the service. This group provides mental health services for
people with ID, neurodevelopmental disorders and services for people with
offending behaviour. Involvement is a challenge because often people within
these care groups have found it hard to engage in mainstream mental health
service user groups. The approach works on two levels of service user and
carer participation.

■ **Level 1.** This is service specific and consists of ward and community groups that are held within the different clinical areas and in community bases, including inpatient and community services for those with ID. Within the services there is some local variation in how user groups are organised, such as who facilitates the group (eg. user-led, staff-led or co-chaired) and the frequency of meetings (some are daily, others weekly). The ID user groups benefit from an external facilitator, and meetings are tailored using various media so that they are accessible to all individuals, thus ensuring participation. These meetings focus on issues surrounding treatment programmes, living together and providing leisure opportunities. Meetings are also minuted, and concerns and issues are fed back to the clinical teams.

■ **Level 2.** This level is made up of users, carers, clinicians and managers, and it reports to the executive. It aims to ensure that the concerns of groups and individuals at service level are heard, and it plans to do this through getting users to gather and provide information, therefore reducing bias of information and encouraging people to come forward. It also works to make improvements, such as the recent development of a new visiting suite.

The entry criteria is that members must have been in a period of recovery for at least six months. This group is also represented by users from all the clinical groups as well as carers and others who have used services from other parts of the organisation.

Many of the user members have had specialist training in a number of areas including cultural competency, staff awareness and running focus groups. This is facilitated by Service Users in Training and Education (SUITE), a user-led training initiative. Others have had experience in talking at conferences about their experiences, while others are experienced auditors of service quality.

The SAINT

In terms of users participating in their own mental health care, the focus in the past has been on reducing symptoms and risk, and to address this we have seen the introduction of the recovery model in mental health care. Recovery is a journey of highs and lows, but it is designed to build resilience and offer hope to people with mental health problems. The aim is not to get people back to where they were before, but to learn from experience and to set goals for the future. Recovery requires a support network of staff, carers and friends that covers all areas affecting mental health. However, how recovery works for people with ID is not clear as their mental health needs and the challenges they face may be different.

Guided self-help (GSH) is an intervention for which user involvement is central to its philosophy. The exact numbers of people with ID who have mental health problems is not known, and in spite of a greater awareness of mental ill-health in people with ID there have been no studies completed that evaluate GSH or interventions to promote mental health. Mental health promotion materials or interventions aimed towards prevention, early detection and helping people cope with mental health problems are in short supply for people with ID, in spite of a number of good mental health promotion leaflets and guides produced for everyday use (Hardy *et al*, 2009).

GSH has been used to help people with, or who are susceptible to, mild depression, and is designed to help people recognise and control the feelings and emotions they are experiencing. However, many available GSH packages often assume a level of cognitive ability and a lifestyle that inadvertently excludes people with ID from using these techniques.

Currently, the SAINT (Chaplin *et al*, 2012), a GSH package designed specifically for people with ID, is being piloted for those vulnerable to poor mental health, and in particular those with symptoms of depression and anxiety. Its aim is to give people control and help them develop strategies for managing mental health problems, and to help those using it identify feelings and emotions they may be experiencing that might threaten their mental well-being. SAINT was developed using both clinical expert opinion and expert service user opinion to produce a GSH tool and training pack. As well as self-help books or manuals, GSH often uses other mediums such as physical exercise (NICE, 2009). SAINT has been produced so that it can be used either independently or with support.

To develop the contents of the SAINT, two established mental health service user groups for people with ID in South London were approached to give their expertise. Ten people from the two groups agreed to take part and they were visited monthly. Three focus groups were conducted, and they were asked to consider and answer the following questions:

1. What activities, interventions or coping skills can help us to feel better about ourselves or help when we are feeling miserable or distressed?

2. How do people feel when they are becoming distressed or mentally unwell? When do we know when we are at risk from becoming unwell?

To help the discussion, examples were given and people were asked to draw on their own personal experiences and knowledge. After each session the user group would send their feedback to a clinical group who were considering the same questions, who in turn would send the user group their answers so that it was available for the next meeting. The aim was to have established a consensus between the two groups by the third meeting, and to have come up with 10 answers for each question. In the last session, a prototype of the SAINT was made available to the user group for comments, which contained the most popular answers thus far. The group was asked for their opinion about the booklet and its accessibility. This included:

- issues of layout
- whether it was easy to understand
- what extra support might be required to use it.

The first focus group generated a total of 40 responses for the first question. The process of agreeing items saw the number reduced to 33. To cut this down further, responses that were similar were merged following agreement from the group eg. 'I feel stress' and 'I feel stressed out'.

For question 1, on coping strategies, there were 58 responses, from which the most popular were compiled into a list, forming the following 10 answers:

1. Speak to someone in your team. This includes having a check-up, taking pills, talking to key workers, seeing a counsellor and calling for a nurse.

2. Speak to someone outside your team who you trust. This includes the Samaritans, family and friends, and someone who can give you the necessary time.

3. Socialise, including day trips or visits to the pub, discos and clubs.

4. Watch TV or DVDs.

5. Listen to music.

6. Keep busy. This includes job hunting, going to classes, using the computer or going shopping.

7. Exercise. This includes sports and activities such as walking.

8. Relax and rest. This includes using a stress ball, breathing exercises, aromatherapy or scented candles, and getting some fresh air.

9. Do or take up a hobby.

10. Read books or find a comforter such as soft toy.

In the second round, the indicators that threaten mental well-being were explored and the various permutations of their answers were merged. Although some do not appear immediately related to mental health, the group was clear that this is how they described certain emotions and feelings.

The top indicators of mental distress or things that threaten mental well-being for the group included:

1. feeling run down; physically unwell; dizzy; in pain.

2. feeling tense; stressed out; uptight.

3. losing appetite.

4. feeling anxious; 'I feel worried'; 'I feel my heart pounding'; 'I feel hot and cold'; 'I feel tingly'; 'I have the shakes'.

5. feeling emotional; upset; experiencing mood swings; heartbroken.

6. feeling strange; 'I don't know who you are'.

7. having problems with sleep; nightmares; waking up; getting out of bed; feeling tired.

8. having a temper; reacting badly to situations.

9. losing concentration.

10. finding it difficult to do things; stopping activities; losing interest in day-to-day life; stopping going out.

In relation to the top coping strategies to promote good mental health, the most popular in round two, following merging, reflected the choices in round one, with the addition of examples to illustrate the statements.

In the last session, a final list of 10 self-reported statements and 10 coping strategies were drawn up. The clinical group were given feedback from the user group and followed a similar process. Finally, accessible language from within the user groups was adopted rather than jargon, for example thought disorder became 'I am having bad thoughts', with examples of what this might mean. Other examples of user-friendly phrases included, 'I am not feeling myself' or 'I feel down today'. All of the statements were backed up by examples such as:

- I feel down today
- I feel sad
- I feel worried
- I feel tense
- I feel stressed
- I find it difficult to do things
- I am losing interest in things
- I don't feel like going out
- I can't be bothered to change my clothes
- I have stopped activities and/or going out.

The process was a learning experience for all involved. As well as establishing ground rules such as listening and not interrupting, people had to agree not to argue with each other's ideas. One such example was the issue of psychotic symptoms, such as hallucinations and delusions. The majority of the groups had no experience of 'voices' or other psychotic phenomena, but some knew people who had experienced this. Using a mixture of explanation and disclosure, most of the group were able to acknowledge that it was distressing to those experiencing it and, in the spirit of making SAINT accessible to people with a wide range of feelings and emotions, the group felt this should be included. In general, the user groups were pragmatic and appeared to concentrate on the vulnerability factors associated with their everyday lives, and focused on the here and now.

In coming to an agreement on coping strategies, the group generated mixed responses. Ideas generated by the group that would normally be considered good advice, such as talking to people to help them with their problem, was not an option for everyone as some people had no one in their lives they could trust. Others said that they would find strategies such as walking away from situations difficult because issues would remain unresolved and they would continue to worry about them. Some were unable to understand how people would enjoy certain activities, such as gardening or exercise. But again, they were willing to accept what others enjoyed and this allowed a wide range of activities to be listed, ensuring that there was likely to be something that appealed to everyone. For many, expressing likes and dislikes was difficult; some found it challenging especially where support was not provided.

The SAINT is still currently in development, and individuals have been recruited to test it out with the aim of establishing whether people with ID can benefit from GSH techniques. For some, the need for more support in order to use it is evident, with those getting the most support doing better. Part of the study seeks to get people's opinions on the approach, regardless of whether it has had any effect in terms of reducing symptom scores.

The SAINT encourages partnerships, and all forms of assessment and treatment should be based upon such partnerships. The reality is that people want to be involved. Some statements follow in the form of a 'bill of rights' that show a desire to be involved and heard. There are many local examples of bills of rights, and the one below was based on the Tuesday Group and Beat the Blues Group (2009), and has been added to by other users.

- We have the right to be treated with respect.
- We have the same rights as any other person.
- We should have the same opportunities as any other person.
- We have the right to make our own decisions.
- We have the right to use the same mental health services as other people.
- We have the right to an advocate if we want one.
- We have the right to be included in all discussions about our mental health.
- We have the right to a wide range of treatments, not just medication.
- We have the right to see what is written about us.

Fred's feedback

Below are some comments from Fred, a 46-year-old man who piloted the SAINT at the time when he was moving from supported living to assisted independent living, having experienced the loss of two people close to him.

How have you found the SAINT?
'I have found it very good and found it very helpful. A lot of people have written down feeling diaries, sad and helpless sort of thing, and this has helped me with my moods as well. I write down how I am feeling. It is a feeling book that helps me with my moods and it has given me the chance to think about my feelings – depressed as well as positive stuff.'

How have you used the SAINT?

'As well as negative stuff, you have to think about the positive stuff because this year has been up and down for me. It's been terrible to start with, but now it is getting better slowly. And I am very proud because there are things like moving, and a new job, and new prospects are coming up for me.'

Is there anything you particularly like about the SAINT?

'The front cover looks like a woman and a man and reminds me of me and my wife and people together. It is very good how it is laid out – I can't read it but it looks understandable. I like the pictures; I am pleased it has pictures in. It helps people with learning disabilities to understand more rather than joined up writing.'

Is there anything you particularly dislike or would change about the SAINT?

'I'll tell you the truth – more pictures for people like myself who cannot read, and for those that can read, more writing and that sort of thing because some people with learning disabilities can read, we all have different things. A guy I know is a good reader so pictures would not be so good for him. I also know guys like Ian who need pictures like the people in my house. The pictures are also good for people learning to read and pick up words.'

When are you most likely to use the SAINT?

'I just use it any time I get depressed, sometimes I use it during the day if I got staff I can talk to. Some staff can be not very understanding but sometimes I get a reasonable member of staff there like my key workers Jill and Roger.

It has helped me sometimes. When I have a good cry I can look at it and say I was depressed or I can say I had a bad day. The next time I could put I had a good day, a nice and happy day. I can also put about my job, so good on one page bad on another.'

Conclusion

This chapter has provided examples of the experiences of people with ID and mood and anxiety disorders, and it has also reported from a user who has participated in piloting GSH techniques designed to equip people with the skills to manage low level symptoms of depression and anxiety. It is clear that people want to be involved their own care and often feel that they are not listened to. To redress this, we have seen how CAG have put systems in place to ensure that the voices of carers and users are heard at all levels of service.

Although this chapter has described some promising pieces of work that promote involvement for users and carers, this is only really the start, and the next step is to empower people with ID to not only be able to access a wider range of interventions but to participate in their development. If we are going to include people in their care, they must be informed in order to make choices for themselves and to manage their own health wherever possible.

Summary

- One easy trap to fall in is to think you know what a person with ID wants and how they are feeling. To avoid this effectively and in an informed way, we need to talk to people as partners in their care.

- User opinion and involvement is vital at all stages of the care process. Input should therefore be visible at all levels of service, from care delivery to the development of new services.

- Partnerships are vital as they allow the person to grow by advocating independence wherever possible. This helps boost self-esteem, reduce stigma and promotes good mental health.

References

Tuesday Group & Beat the Blues Group (2009) It's our mental health. *Advances in Mental Health and Learning Disabilities* **3** (2) 40–41.

Chaplin E, Bouras N & Craig T (2012) Using service user and clinical opinion to develop the SAINT: A guided self-help pack for adults with intellectual disability. *Advances in Mental Health and Intellectual Disabilities* **6** (1) 17–25.

Cole A (2002) *Include Us Too: Developing and improving services to meet the mental health needs of people with learning disabilities*. London: IAHSP.

Department of Health (2001) *Nothing About Us Without Us*. London: TSO.

Department of Health (2009) *Valuing People Now*. London: TSO.

Department of Health (2011) *No Health Without Mental Health*. London: Central Office of Information.

Department of Health and Social Security (2005) *Equal Lives: Review of policy and services for people with a learning disability in Northern Ireland*. Belfast: DHSSPS.

Estia Centre (2003) *Our Mental Health: A report by the Tuesday Group*. London: Estia Centre.

Foundation for People with Learning Disabilities (2004) *Green Light For Mental Health: How good are your mental health services for people with learning disabilities? A service improvement toolkit*. London: Foundation for People with Learning Disabilities.

National Institute of Health and Clinical Excellence (NICE) (2009) *Depression: The treatment and management of depression in adults (update) Clinical Guidelines CG90*. London: NICE.

Hardy S, Woodward P, Halls S & Creet B (2009) *Mental Health Promotion for People with Learning Disabilities*. Brighton: Pavilion.

Welsh Office (2001) *Fulfilling the Promises*. Cardiff: Welsh Office.

Chapter 5

Case formulation

Barry Ingham

Overview

This chapter will outline the use of case formulation in working with people with ID who experience anxiety and depression. In particular, it will examine the role that case formulation plays within a broader biopsychosocial model and its application to the systems that support people with ID. It will also outline a protocol for workshops that develop collaborative case formulations in order to help staff who work with people with ID, and provide a fictional case study about an individual experiencing anxiety and depression in the context of these workshops, to demonstrate how the workshops may act as interventions. The change techniques used within the case formulation development process will be demonstrated alongside a discussion of the outcomes associated with the case formulation approach.

Learning objectives

■ Provide a definition of case formulation and describe its role in people with ID and anxiety or depression.

■ Be aware of the protocol used for case formulation development workshops, and the change techniques used within this.

■ Consider the potential links between case formulation and outcome.

Introduction

Case formulation is considered central to psychological healthcare and to evidence based psychological therapies for anxiety and depression in mainstream populations (eg. talking therapies such as cognitive behavioural therapy (CBT) (Beck, 1995)). It is defined as the collation of assessment information integrated with theory and practice in order to provide an explanation or individual clinical theory that accounts for the development and maintenance of the presenting problems, and then guides interventions to manage those problems (Tarrier & Calam, 2002). The evidence base for case formulation's role in psychological therapies is emerging (Kuyken *et al*, 2008) and its application to broader psychological processes, such as coping with stress, is being considered (Johnston *et al*, 2011). In addition, its use at a systemic, organisational level to help understand and manage complex presentations is developing, for example within mainstream inpatient services (Berry *et al*, 2009). Case formulation is also seen as a key competence within UK mental healthcare professions such as clinical psychology (Division of Clinical Psychology, 2010) and psychiatry (Royal College of Psychiatrists, 2010).

Case formulation for people with ID

It is now widely acknowledged that approaches to mental healthcare for people with ID (including anxiety and depression) should be psychosocial, integrated and multidisciplinary (Dagnan, 2007), however the evidence base remains limited and further work is required to establish approaches that work (Gustafsson *et al*, 2009). Hatton and Taylor (2005) suggest following mainstream mental health services, whereby biological, psychological and social approaches are provided in an integrated manner ie. using a biopsychosocial model (Engel, 1980). Biopsychosocial approaches encourage the use of multidisciplinary case formulation to integrate different aspects of clinical information, explain the development and maintenance of problems and then guide appropriate interventions to address those problems (Kinderman & Tai, 2006). The interventions selected by the formulation may then be managed by different members of the multidisciplinary care team according to the biological, psychological or social nature of the intervention (Kinderman & Tai, 2006). With this in mind, there has been some application of biopsychosocial approaches to ID inpatient services (Isherwood *et al*, 2004; Ingham & Clarke, 2009), and the further development of these approaches within services for people with ID may help to improve their quality and meet the complex needs of this client group.

In terms of talking therapies, the use of case formulation as a key feature of CBT for people with ID is increasingly recommended (Dagnan, 2007; Jahoda *et al*, 2009). There are also specific examples of using formulation within psychological therapies for people with ID who experience psychotic symptoms (Kirkland, 2005), anger problems (Willner, 2009) and display challenging behaviour (British Psychological Society, 2004). However, this chapter will focus on the use of case formulation as a central feature of biopsychosocial approaches to managing anxiety and depression. It will also focus on applying this to the systems around individuals with ID who have experienced anxiety and depression that was sufficiently severe to require inpatient admission.

Case formulation for anxiety and depression in ID

People with ID may experience an increased vulnerability to mental health problems, and prevalence studies indicate that problems such as anxiety are common within this population (Reid *et al*, 2011). Studies have also indicated biopsychosocial factors associated with the development and maintenance of anxiety and depression in people with ID. For example, historical factors, such as traumatic life events, may predispose individuals to experiencing current anxiety symptoms (Wigham *et al*, 2011). Kiddle and Dagnan (2011) suggest that developmental factors interacting with the individual's social environment could contribute to the likelihood of people with ID experiencing depression.

Contemporary factors, such as current demands upon social skills and resources in unstructured environments, may also influence the maintenance of anxiety problems (Einfeld *et al*, 2006). Furthermore, Hartley and McLean (2009) found that negative self-appraisals and dysfunctional coping strategies were more likely in depressed than non-depressed groups of people with ID. These, and a range of other factors, indicate the complexity involved in understanding, treating and managing anxiety and depression, particularly where people experience additional communication impairments and there is a requirement for specialist, paid carer support. Dagnan (2007) suggests that key psychosocial factors involved in anxiety and depression, such as social context and cognitive functioning, could be integrated through psychosocial case formulations in order to better understand these complex difficulties.

Case formulation workshops

One of the important principles of case formulation is that it is developed collaboratively with those involved in the presenting problems (Kuyken *et al,* 2008). In talking therapies, such as CBT, this is often a collaborative development with the referred individual in a one-to-one setting. However, people with ID who also experience anxiety and depression may require high levels of staff support, whose role may be to provide support for adaptive functioning impairments. They are also likely to provide additional emotional and social support and so may be important in managing (or maintaining) psychosocial difficulties. For this population then, collaborative case formulation development with staff could help them internalise a more adequate explanation or attribution of the presenting difficulties and so improve their support and management while reducing the likelihood of maintaining those difficulties. Attempts have been made to help staff teams understand and respond to psychosocial difficulties displayed by people with ID (eg. Gentry *et al,* 2001), and while these have tended to focus on managing severe challenging behaviour, they may also be applied to problems such as anxiety and depression.

A protocol has been developed that uses a workshop format and the principles of case formulation development alongside the use of systemic techniques. This approach centres on developing a formulation based on a thorough understanding, and a collaboratively developed hypothesis, of an individual's psychosocial difficulties, that covers five different areas. These areas, known as the 'five Ps', are as follows.

1. **Presenting issues or problems.** What are the current problems the person faces, primarily in terms of difficult behaviours, emotions and thoughts? It is important to describe these problems in a detailed and individual way. The development of a problem list is considered to be a way of determining short, medium and long-term goals.

2. **Predisposing factors.** Aspects that contribute to the origins and development of the problems should be analysed and noted. There is an emphasis here on considering historical events, both internal and external, and the quantity and quality of these events in relation to the individual ie. a large number of difficult past events could have a significant impact, but the meaning of those past events for the individual is also important.

3. **Precipitating factors.** Recent external and internal factors that have led to the presenting problems being experienced now should be identified. These events can be external (eg. time or place) or internal (eg. thoughts or feelings).

4. **Perpetuating factors.** In order to come to a case formulation, the factors that are keeping the presenting problems going should be considered and maintenance cycles for the current problems, such as those seen in panic and phobias, should be identified.

5. **Protective factors.** The workshops should also aim to identify the strengths and resiliencies that the person can draw on in order to manage and prevent the problems from escalating, including coping strategies and social networks.

(Ingham *et al*, 2008).

The longitudinal and holistic view of an individual and their difficulties that is gathered in this way can then be used to guide interventions by identifying key factors that could be built upon or changed, for example, to build on existing functional coping strategies or to break unhelpful cycles of stress. An action plan can then be developed consisting of these interventions, which would be implemented and reviewed and, if necessary, the formulation (and subsequent interventions) would be changed on the basis of this.

How the workshops work

A protocol for the use of collaborative case formulation development workshops (using the five Ps approach) has been developed and initially evaluated (Ingham, 2011a). These workshops involve staff supporting individuals with ID who display psychosocial difficulties, including anxiety and depression, that risk placement breakdown and admission to inpatient services. The workshops have been designed to use the five Ps framework over two sessions of three hours to collaboratively develop a case formulation with staff to help explain the occurrence, and guide management, of psychosocial difficulties.

Each workshop is attended by the relevant staff involved in a case, and is facilitated by a clinical psychologist or similarly qualified professional. A comprehensive notes review is completed before the first workshop, which consists of historical information about the person, ordered into different sections, such as history of mental health difficulties, family history and psychological assessments. In addition, the notes review contains a timeline of significant life events. This review is presented at the start of the first workshop and read by staff in order to increase awareness of the historical factors that may impact upon presenting problems. The initial discussions in the first workshop and the connections between the various elements of the case that were identified by the notes review serve as the starting point for the development of a formulation.

The workshops are then structured to provide information on what a formulation entails and each of the different aspects of a five Ps formulation listed earlier are considered in depth. After one particular aspect of the five Ps formulation has been described, the facilitator helps staff to explore the various important issues within that aspect. Towards the end of the process, the different aspects of the five Ps formulation are integrated by the facilitator and the staff.

Recommendations for support and interventions would then be developed by the team on the basis of the formulation.

Case study: Alison

Alison is an individual with ID living alone in an urban area who had been presenting with significant anxiety and low mood. She had a history of alcohol misuse and had attempted suicide by taking an overdose. It was therefore necessary to admit her to an acute mental health ID inpatient service. She had a chaotic family life and was inconsistent in the use of health and social care services that had been put in place to help support her mental health difficulties. There was increasing worry surrounding Alison's physical health due to the overdoses and alcohol misuse, and she had, for example, developed diabetes. A comprehensive notes review and assessment highlighted a history of difficulties with her mood and a transient lifestyle, interacting with specific cognitive impairment (including executive functioning impairments) and experiences of bullying, prejudice and a feeling of failure throughout life.

The collaborative case formulation development workshops were held following an inpatient admission and, in terms of the five Ps, Alison's case formulation was as follows:

- Presenting issues or problems:
  - low mood and anxiety (emotions)
  - negative views of self as a failure and isolated (thoughts)
  - attempted suicide (eg. overdose) and alcohol misuse (behaviours).

- Predisposing factors:
  - specific cognitive impairment, with problems in executive functioning (eg. planning and understanding consequences)

- experience of stigma and bullying from childhood (eg. receiving special education)
- criticism from family members throughout life, except from her mother who died recently
- traumatic experiences including physical and sexual assault
- an interaction of the above may have led to negative self-evaluation and social comparison that developed the belief that she was a bad person who others weren't able to understand or help. As such, she had developed dysfunctional ways of coping with stress eg. alcohol misuse.

- **Precipitating factors:**
  - trusted individuals leaving or being unavailable (eg. community nurse)
  - removal of support services due to Alison reporting she did not require them
  - drinking large amounts of alcohol in order to cope with low mood and isolation
  - family members becoming over-involved with her life (eg. wanting to move in with her)
  - stressful situations didn't necessarily lead to alcohol use/overdose – it may be that this was mediated by underlying factors, such as whether Alison perceived herself as failing or isolated.

- **Perpetuating factors:**
  - Alison often perceived that no one understood her and that she was the only one that she could rely on, which led to self-isolation when stressed
  - when she drank excessively, she would feel shame and guilt and try to hide this from others
  - due to low self-esteem and a reluctance to ask for help for fear of upsetting others, she would often tell key health and social care professionals that everything was fine despite experiencing low mood and suicidal thoughts
  - Alison had limited coping skills due to cognitive impairments, which meant that she often struggled to estimate consequences and plan ways of seeking support
  - when Alison's family members were aware of increasing difficulties they would often criticise her to try and get her to change. She found this particularly difficult, which maintained low self-esteem and dysfunctional coping strategies. In this way, Alison's mental health difficulties and family criticism maintained each other.

- Protective factors:
  - Alison was able to advocate for herself, express her own needs and be involved in planning for the future if given appropriate support to do so
  - when engaged in occupation and a fulfilling caring role with others, Alison's mood often lifted and engagement in dysfunctional coping methods reduced
  - Alison was able to develop valued trusting relationships with others, but needed support to maintain these during stressful times
  - she had her own house and valued the independence this gave her, which boosted her self-esteem.

This case formulation indicated that Alison's long-standing experience of anxiety and depression was underpinned by shame, guilt and low self-esteem. These difficulties had developed over time through a range of biopsychosocial factors, and they were likely to continue without ongoing, structured support. This analysis guided interventions and the creation of an action plan, which included individual work while Alison was an inpatient that could also be continued upon discharge (eg. CBT to develop more functional coping skills to cope with low mood), and systemic work for planning discharge (eg. development of a multidisciplinary, biopsychosocial relapse management plan).

On the basis of this formulation, the following action plan was devised:

- Share, develop and reformulate the above formulation with Alison to check validity and to facilitate a better understanding of her difficulties.
- Undertake CBT with Alison to include self-esteem development while she was an inpatient, and continue these principles when she returns home to develop more appropriate coping strategies.
- Offer family therapy to Alison's family members to reduce criticism on discharge.
- Develop a discharge plan based on the formulation for all staff involved with Alison, including:
  - upon returning to living on her own, aim to maintain independence but with more regular and frequent support that is not reduced without careful review
  - create a relapse management plan where the early warning signs of increased anxiety/depression are detected and responded to in order to reduce likelihood of readmission
  - regular multidisciplinary review of the plan once Alison is discharged to ensure that it is still meeting her needs.

This action plan shifted the staff's perception and behaviour towards Alison away from attempts to eliminate her difficulties and towards planning to provide structured support that would help her to self-regulate. Inherent in this was an acknowledgement from staff that Alison would continue to struggle in managing her difficulties independently, but that a collaborative approach should be taken that would allow her to retain significant control over everyday decisions and activities. This biopsychosocial model of ongoing support (as opposed to a model of identifying treatment in order to cure) facilitated Alison's discharge and she was able to retain her independence without requiring readmission to hospital.

After the formulation development process with staff, it was agreed that the formulation should be shared and further developed with Alison as part of the ongoing treatment plan. However, it was agreed that an abridged version of the formulation should be the starting point for this and that it should be checked with Alison as valid and understandable. Alison received this positively and she used the abridged version as a reference point within the relapse management plan developed for discharge.

Techniques and principles used within the workshops and their impact on staff

A number of processes aiming to change the understanding of staff and increase their empathy for, and confidence in, Alison (in order that these might act as potential mediators for her anxiety and depression) were facilitated through the workshop. This included approaches taken from family or systemic therapy that were then adapted and applied to working with families and care staff teams supporting people with ID (Rikberg Smyly, 2009). Family and systemic therapies use a framework of understanding where people and problems are formed within relationships. Systemic techniques are then used to explore patterns and stories within these relationships with the aim of eliciting change within staff teams.

One such technique is the use of circular questioning (Penn, 1982), whereby care staff are asked questions about how others (including the person they are supporting) think or feel in order to generate information about interactions and to allow individuals to reflect on their (possibly dysfunctional) role in those relationships. For example, discussion within the above workshop highlighted that Alison experienced a greater sense of guilt, shame and anxiety where she perceived herself to have failed. At the same time, others (including staff) had not actively supported her in considering alternative perspectives or applying more functional coping strategies because she was reluctant to seek help at those times.

In the workshop, the anxiety resulting from shame experienced by Alison was explored by considering the ways in which she interacted with others and how staff responded to her (eg. by not responding proactively at times when Alison perceived she had failed and started to self-isolate or reject help from others). Staff often responded to Alison by allowing her the 'choice' of avoiding support from others. This may then have confirmed her negative self-image and increased the likelihood of engaging in dysfunctional coping strategies, thus maintaining or exacerbating her anxiety and guilt.

Alison's lack of capacity to make such a decision, therefore, particularly when she is more anxious or depressed, led to an agreement that decisions about support should be made proactively by staff (with Alison's advance agreement). Staff responses to Alison should then be clear, consistent and predictably related to need (leading to the development of a relapse management plan shared by Alison and the staff). Circular questioning within the context of formulation development helped to reach this new understanding and to develop a plan.

Key principles within CBT were also applied throughout this process, such as collaborative empiricism (ie. sharing information and testing out ideas jointly) and Socratic questioning (ie. to enable guided discovery) (Beck, 1995). For example, staff were not directly provided with a formulation or a plan to meet Alison's needs. Instead, the facilitator encouraged them to examine data and evidence around Alison's coping strategies, intellectual functioning and mental health difficulties, and then to develop a strategy for therapeutic support and regulation based on an individual explanation of her difficulties. This was implemented and reviewed to support her following discharge.

These techniques (collaborative empiricism and Socratic questioning) have been the driving force behind the developing evidence base of CBT in addressing anxiety and depression in mainstream populations, and there have been previous attempts to apply them to staff supporting individuals with ID (Kushlick et al, 1997). A collaborative, 'not knowing' approach was also taken by the facilitator, and, for example, staff were the experts when it came to providing information about Alison, and they were encouraged to challenge each other and the facilitator about important factors related to her difficulties.

These techniques were used as the guiding principles by the facilitator within the workshop format with the aim of constructing a formulation that would enable and guide a more appropriate management of the anxiety and depression experienced by Alison, and using these techniques and principles may have helped staff to develop a more adequate explanation for the problems that Alison presented with.

For Alison and the staff team around her, formulation development may prove to be a valuable framework for helping address anxiety and depression symptoms through problem solving and developing optimism and confidence when faced with complex problems. The change techniques involved (eg. guided discovery to develop new understandings) may act as potential mediators of anxiety and depression (such as emotional responses from staff) and so help manage anxiety and depression, thereby supporting discharge and preventing readmission to inpatient services.

While Alison's case was set within a specific clinical context, it is likely that the principles and techniques used could be applied to a range of problems and contexts with individuals and systems.

Case study outcomes

Psychosocial assessments may be used to indicate outcomes following case formulation development workshops. Potential measures include measures of anxiety (the Glasgow Anxiety Scale) (Mindham & Espie, 2003), depression (Glasgow Depression Scale) (Cuthill, Espie & Cooper, 2003) and self-esteem (Culture Free Self Esteem Inventory) (Battle, 1992) specifically developed or adapted for people with ID.

Figure 5.1 summarises these measures as completed by Alison, and indicates that she was experiencing less anxiety and depression and reported higher self-esteem following the formulation development process. Furthermore, Alison was discharged with an action plan as guided by the formulation and did not require a readmission.

Figure 5.1: Changes in measures of anxiety, depression and self-esteem following formulation development workshops

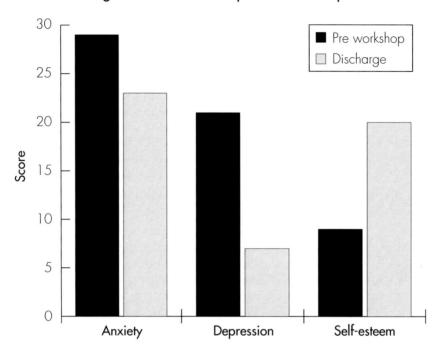

This demonstrates one way of examining outcomes related to case formulation development. However, more work needs to be done in this area to provide evidence for the link between formulation and outcomes.

Potential outcomes related to case formulation development

There are a number of things that one might expect to change through the formulation process as described above. The end goal is to establish a link between formulation and changes in a client's quality of life (ideally, an improvement). However, the link between case formulation and outcome in mainstream therapeutic approaches has been difficult to establish (Kuyken *et al*, 2008). This may be because there are a number of mediating/moderating factors between the development of a case formulation and the final outcome (eg. the expertise of the person developing the formulation, the validity of the formulation produced or the implementation of interventions based on the formulation).

As a result, a range of approaches to examining changes following formulation workshops have been developed, including exploring the change processes that take place within systems during a formulation workshop. Staff involved with formulation development workshops have previously been asked to give their views on the change mechanisms occurring, and they report that the workshops enabled them to share new information about the individual. It also altered their thinking about the individual and focused their goals for working with them (Ingham & Clarke, 2009). This fits with Tarrier and Calam's (2002) definition of case formulation, noted earlier, and if these changes are occurring then it may follow that more appropriate interventions will take place. This should increase the likelihood of quicker and more significant improvements in mental health.

However, there are also a number of factors that help or hinder these change processes, such as ensuring that the process is sufficiently collaborative and that certain key individuals are involved. Care should therefore be taken that these things are addressed throughout this process if positive outcomes are to occur.

There has also been some evidence for changes in knowledge, confidence and empathy reported by staff in relation to the client, and they also report that they are able to say more about the client and their difficulties after completing a formulation workshop (Ingham, 2011b). Again, these changes would be expected precursors to a more accurate, consistent and positive response to the client.

Conclusion

This chapter has outlined the role of case formulation in understanding and intervening in anxiety and depression experienced by people with ID, particularly in using a biopsychosocial model to make sense of the complexity that is associated with this population, and in developing a plan to help manage their difficulties. The specific application of collaborative case formulation development workshops may be a framework to achieve this. In Alison's case, these workshops enabled the system around her to develop a better understanding of her needs, and this guided a more appropriate plan to help her. However, more work is required to explore the link between case formulation development and outcome.

It is clear, however, that the use of formulation should be considered and evaluated when developing ways in which individuals with ID, and the systems supporting them, are helped to manage anxiety and depression.

Summary

- Case formulation for people with ID and anxiety or depression aims to provide an individual, theoretical explanation for the development and maintenance of presenting problems, and aims to guide biopsychosocial interventions to manage those problems.

- Collaborative case formulation development workshops have been constructed to help care staff to develop case formulations for individuals with ID.

- Through the development of a case formulation, these workshops may help to change unhelpful attributions, emotions and behaviours from staff in relation to the individual they support.

- Development of a case formulation may be associated with improved outcomes for individuals with ID who are also experiencing anxiety or depression.

References

Battle J (1992) *Culture-Free Self-Esteem Inventories* (2nd edition). Austin, TX: Pro-Ed.

Beck J (1995) *Cognitive Therapy: Basics and beyond*. New York: Guilford.

Berry K, Barrowclough C & Wearden A (2009) A pilot study investigating the use of psychological formulations to modify psychiatric staff perceptions of service users with psychosis. *Behavioural and Cognitive Psychotherapy* **37** (1) 39–48.

British Psychological Society (2004) *Psychological Interventions for Severely Challenging Behaviours Shown by People with Learning Disabilities*. Leicester: The British Psychological Society.

Cuthill F, Espie C & Cooper S (2003) Development and psychometric properties of the Glasgow Depression Scale for people with a learning disability. *British Journal of Psychiatry* **182** 347–353.

Dagnan D (2007) Psychosocial interventions for people with learning disabilities. *Advances in Mental Health and Learning Disabilities* **1** (2) 3–7.

Division of Clinical Psychology (2010) *The Core Purpose and Philosophy of the Profession*. Leicester: The British Psychological Society.

Einfeld S, Piccinin A, Mackinnon A, Hofer S, Taffe J, Gray K, Bontempo D, Hoffman L, Parmenter T & Tonge B (2006) Psychopathology in young people with intellectual disability. *Journal of the American Medical Association* **296** (16) 1981–1989.

Engel G (1980) The clinical application of the biopsychosocial model. *American Journal of Psychiatry* **137** 535–544.

Gentry M, Iceton J & Milne D (2001) Managing challenging behaviour in the community: methods and results of interactive staff training. *Health & Social Care in the Community* **9** (3) 143–150.

Gustafsson C, Ojehagen A, Hansson L, Sandlund M, Nystrom M, Glad J, Cruce G, Jonsson A & Fredriksson M (2009) Effects of psychosocial interventions for people with intellectual disabilities and mental health problems: a survey of systematic reviews. *Research on Social Work Practice* **19** (3) 281–290.

Hatton C & Taylor J (2005) Promoting healthy lifestyles: mental health and illness. In: G Grant, P Goward, M Richardson and P Ramcharan (Eds) *Learning Disability: A life cycle approach to valuing people*. Maidenhead: Open University Press.

Hartley S & McLean W (2009) Depression in adults with mild intellectual disability: role of stress, attributions, and coping. *American Journal on Intellectual and Developmental Disabilities* **114** (3) 147–160.

Ingham B (2011a) Collaborative psychosocial case formulation development workshops: a case study with direct care staff. *Advances in Mental Health and Intellectual Disabilities* **5** (2) 9–15.

Ingham B (2011b) *Collaborative psychosocial formulation in intellectual/developmental disabilities: What difference does it make?* Presentation at the British Association of Behavioural and Cognitive Psychotherapies Annual Conference, Guildford.

Ingham B, Clarke L & James I (2008) Biopsychosocial case formulation for people with intellectual disabilities and mental health problems: a pilot study of a training workshop for direct care staff. *British Journal of Developmental Disabilities* **54** (1) 41–54.

Ingham B & Clarke L (2009) The introduction of clinical psychology services to an inpatient autistic spectrum disorders and intellectual disabilities service: impact and reflections. *Clinical Psychology Forum* **106** 41–54.

Isherwood T, Burns M & Rigby G (2004) Psychosocial interventions in a medium secure unit for people with learning disabilities: a service development. *Mental Health and Learning Disabilities Research and Practice* **1** (1) 29–35.

Jahoda A, Dagnan D, Stenfert-Kroese B, Pert C & Trower P (2009) Cognitive behavioural therapy: from face to face interaction to a broader contextual understanding of change. *Journal of Intellectual Disabilities Research* **53** (9) 759–771.

Johnston L, Hutchison A & Ingham B (2011) The utility of biopsychosocial models of clinical formulation within stress and coping theory and applied practice. In: T Davenport (Ed) *Managing Stress: From theory to practice*. New York: Nova Publishers.

Kiddle H & Dagnan D (2011) Vulnerability to depression in adolescents with intellectual disabilities. *Advances in Mental Health and Intellectual Disabilities* **5** (1) 3–8.

Kinderman P & Tai S (2006) Clinical implications of a psychological model of mental disorder. *Behavioural and Cognitive Psychotherapy* **35** 1–14.

Kirkland J (2005) Cognitive-behaviour formulation for three men with learning disabilities who experience psychosis: how do we make it make sense? *British Journal of Learning Disabilities* **33** (4) 160–165.

Kushlick A, Trower P & Dagnan D (1997) Applying cognitive behavioural approaches to the carers of people with learning disabilities. In: B Kroese, D Dagnan & K Loumides (Eds) *Cognitive Behaviour Therapy for People with Learning Disabilities*. London: Routledge.

Kuyken W, Padesky C & Dudley R (2008) The science and practice of case conceptualisation. *Behavioural and Cognitive Psychotherapy* **36** (6) 757–768.

Mindham J & Espie C (2003) Glasgow anxiety scale for people with an intellectual disability (GAS-ID): development and psychometric properties of a new measure for use with people with mild intellectual disability. *Journal of Intellectual Disability Research* **47** (Pt1) 22–30.

Penn P (1982) Circular questioning. *Family Process* **21** 267–280.

Reid K, Smiley E & Cooper S (2011) Prevalence and associations of anxiety disorders in adults with intellectual disabilities. *Journal of Intellectual Disability Research* **55** (2) 172–181.

Rikberg Smyly S (2009) Working systemically with people with learning disabilities. In: H Beinart, P Kennedy & S Llewelyn (Eds) *Clinical Psychology in Practice*. Chichester: John Wiley & Sons.

Royal College of Psychiatrists (2010) A competency based curriculum for specialist core training in psychiatry [online]. London: Royal College of Psychiatrists. Available at: http://www.rcpsych.ac.uk/training/curriculum2010.aspx (accessed March 2012)

Tarrier N & Calam R (2002) New developments in cognitive-behavioural case formation. Epidemiological, systemic and social context: an integrative approach. *Behavioural and Cognitive Psychotherapy* **30** (3) 311–328.

Wigham S, Taylor J & Hatton C (2011) The effects of traumatizing life events on people with intellectual disabilities: a systematic review. *Journal of Mental Health Research in Intellectual Disabilities* **4** (1) 19–39.

Willner P (2009) A cognitive-behavioural formulation of anger in a man with an intellectual disability. In: P Sturmey (Ed) *Clinical Case Formulation: Varieties of Approaches*. Chichester: John Wiley & Sons.

Chapter 6

Psychopharmacological approaches

Caroline Reid and Shoumitro Deb

Overview

This chapter provides an overview on the pharmacological (medicinal) management of anxiety and depression in people with ID. It discusses the national guidelines on treating these disorders and modifications that may need to be made for people with ID. It also summarises the available evidence from the literature on pharmacological management of anxiety and depression in this population.

Learning objectives

- To understand the general principles of prescribing medication for people with ID.
- To have a knowledge of the medication that can be used to treat depression and anxiety in people with ID.
- To understand the 'stepped' management approach to treating depression and anxiety in people with ID.

General principles

Overall, the guidelines provided by NICE for the use of medication for anxiety and depression apply to people with ID. However, it is important to consider certain issues when prescribing medication for this group. As some people with ID have communication difficulties, it may be difficult to ascertain if the medication is helping the patient or if they are having any adverse effects (Bhaumik & Branford, 2008). A person's ID will also impact on their capacity to consent to treatment. Capacity must be assessed when prescribing medication, with every effort made to provide people with ID with accessible information to help them with their decision. There are accessible versions (easy read) of information leaflets available with accompanying audio versions for people with ID and their carers to download from the internet (www.ld-medication.bham.ac.uk) (Unwin & Deb, 2006). A person with ID and their carer should be fully consulted when taking any decision about prescribing medication (Hall & Deb, 2008).

Guidance checklists for prescribing medication to people with ID, such as the one that follows, are available from national and international guidelines:

- always assess a person's capacity to consent to treatment
- start with a low dose
- when increasing the dose of medication, do so gradually
- ensure clear instructions are given to the patient and carer about why they are taking the medication and how to take it
- clearly state the outcomes that would indicate a benefit from taking the medication, so the patient and carers can look out for these
- be vigilant in looking for side effects
- review medication regularly
- be aware of other medication the person is taking that may interact with the medication you wish to prescribe
- be aware of co-morbid medical conditions, such as epilepsy, which may be affected by the medication you wish to prescribe
- the person prescribing the medication should identify a key person who will ensure that the medication is administered appropriately, and communicate all changes to the relevant parties.

(Deb *et al*, 2006; Deb *et al*, 2009; Unwin & Deb, 2010; Banks *et al*, 2007)

NICE guidelines follow a 'stepped' approach to care in which the first suggested step in any treatment is the least intrusive and most effective. If a person does not respond to this step, or does not wish to receive the treatment at this step, then the clinician should move up to the next step.

Management of depression

The management of depression includes a comprehensive assessment and diagnosis followed by treatment by competent practitioners in either a psychological or pharmacological approach, or a combination of these. A stepped approach for the management of depression, as suggested by the most recent NICE guidelines, is as follows (NICE, 2009) (see Table 6.1).

Table 6.1: A stepped approach to managing depression

Step 1:	All known and suspected presentations of depression.
	Assessment, support, psycho-education, active monitoring and referral for further assessment and monitoring.
Step 2:	Persistent sub-threshold depressive symptoms, mild–moderate depression.
	Low intensity psychological and psychosocial interventions, medication and referral for further assessment and interventions.
Step 3:	Persistent sub-threshold depressive symptoms, mild–moderate depression with inadequate response to initial interventions, or moderate–severe depression.
	Medication, high intensity psychological interventions, combined treatments, collaborative care and referral for further assessment and interventions.
Step 4:	Severe and complex depression, risk to life, severe self-neglect.
	Medications, high intensity psychological treatment, electroconvulsive therapy, crisis service, combined treatments, multi-professional and inpatient care.

Medications for the management of depression

There are many different theories on the aetiology of depression, including genetic theories, early childhood experiences, personality and social environment. It is believed that whatever the cause, there is ultimately a change in the chemicals in the brain that creates the clinical symptoms of depression. The main chemicals involved are called 'monoamine neurotransmitters', two of which that have a particular involvement in depression are called 'serotonin' and 'noradrenaline'. It is said that in depression there are low levels of these monoamine neurotransmitters in the brain, and this forms the basis of how antidepressant medications are used to treat depression, as they work to increase these levels (Gelder *et al*, 2006).

Choice of antidepressant

The NICE guidelines state that any choice of antidepressant should be discussed with the patient. This should include a consideration of all potential adverse effects, the effect of stopping the medication, potential interactions with other medications that the person is taking simultaneously or other health problems that they also have, and their perception of the effectiveness and tolerability of any other antidepressants they have previously received. In a person who has an ID this needs to be tailored to their individual needs, with every attempt made to provide accessible information for them and their carers (Unwin & Deb, 2006).

Selective serotonin re-uptake inhibitors

The first choice of antidepressant is a family/class called selective serotonin re-uptake inhibitors (SSRIs). This group of medications works by stopping the monoamine neurotransmitter serotonin being taken up by the nerve endings in the brain, and thus increasing the levels of serotonin in the brain. The reason SSRIs are the first choice antidepressant is because there is good evidence that they are as effective as other classes of antidepressants and they have a better risk/benefit balance regarding their adverse effects than other classes of antidepressant medications. They are also less dangerous in overdose than the older generation of antidepressants (Gelder *et al*, 2006).

The SSRIs currently licensed for the management of depression are citalopram, escitalopram, fluoexetine, fluvoxamine, paroxetine and sertraline (see Table 6.2 on p110).

There are, however, some issues that need to be considered when using SSRIs:

■ SSRIs may increase the frequency of seizures or reduce the threshold at which seizures occur in people with epilepsy. They should therefore be used with caution in patients with propensity to develop epileptic seizures. This is of particular relevance in people with ID as there is a higher proportion of people with epilepsy in this population as compared with people without ID (Deb, 2007; Berney & Deb, 2012).

■ SSRIs can increase the risk of bleeding. They should, therefore, be used with caution in people who are on other medications that also increase the risk of bleeding (such as warfarin or non-steroidal anti-inflammatory drugs (NSAIDs)) or who have a history of bleeding disorders (especially gastrointestinal bleeding).

■ SSRIs should be used with caution in people with cardiac disease, diabetes mellitus or a susceptibility to angle-closure glaucoma.

The adverse effects of SSRIs are:

■ Nausea, vomiting, indigestion, abdominal pain, diarrhoea, constipation, reduced appetite and weight loss.

■ Increased levels of anxiety and agitation. This may be particularly difficult for individuals with ID who are not able to express their distress verbally. This usually settles after a few weeks of being on the medication.

■ Possible increased thoughts of self-harm, and suicidal thoughts and acts when initiating treatment.

■ Sexual dysfunction, including reduced interest in sexual activity.

■ Difficulty sleeping.

■ Urinary retention (being unable to pass urine).

■ Sweating.

■ Tremors.

■ Rash.

■ Low sodium levels in the blood (hyponatraemia).

Withdrawal from SSRIs

Stopping SSRIs abruptly can cause a withdrawal reaction, and so should be done slowly and gradually. This withdrawal reaction is worst with paroxetine. Symptoms include:

■ headache

■ anxiety

■ dizziness

■ sleep disturbance

■ electric shock sensations

Table 6.2: SSRIs: Guideline according to the Maudsley Prescribing Guideline (Taylor et al, 2007)

SSRI	Licensed dose	Main adverse effects	Main interactions
Citalopram	20–40mg a day. Recent evidence suggests that doses over 40 mgs a day can cause problems with the heart. Maximum dose for use among elderly people is 20 mgs a day.	As listed on page 109.	Avoid using with St John's Wort, monoamine oxidase inhibitors (MAOIs) and medications that increase risk of bleeding.
Escitalopram (This is very similar to citalopram but is more expensive)	10–20mg a day.	As listed on page 109.	As for citalopram.
Fluoxetine	20–60mg a day.	As listed on page 109 but sleeping difficulties and agitation may be more common. Rash may occur more frequently. People with diabetes mellitus may need their insulin regimen altered.	Can increase blood levels of some antipsychotics, benzodiazepines, carbamazepine and Tricyclic antidepressants (TCAs). Should never be used with MAOIs. Avoid St John's Wort and medications that increase risk of bleeding.
Fluvoxamine	100–300mg a day. Not often used.	As listed on page 109 but nausea more common.	As for fluoxetine.
Paroxetine	20–50mg a day. Evidence for higher doses is poor.	As listed on page 109 but sedation, urinary problems and tremor more common. Discontinuation symptoms common.	As for fluoxetine.
Sertraline	50–200mg a day. There is poor evidence for higher doses.	As above.	As for fluoxetine.

- sweating
- flu-like symptoms
- sensory symptoms such as numbness and a feeling of 'pins and needles'.

Investigations

No specific investigations are needed at baseline (before starting the medication) or for monitoring. Investigation is only needed if the person develops adverse effects that indicate a certain investigation needs to be carried out, for example, a blood test to check sodium levels if a person presents with symptoms of low sodium.

Tricyclic antidepressants

Tricyclic antidepressants (TCAs) are an older class of antidepressant medications that work by reducing the uptake of the monoamine neurotransmitters serotonin and noradrenaline, therefore increasing their levels in the brain. Examples of TCAs include amitriptyline, clomipramine, dosulepin, doxepin, imipramine, lofepramine, nortriptyline and trimipramine (Joint Formulary Committee, 2011) (see Table 6.3 on p113).

There are certain issues that need to be considered when using TCAs:

- They should be used with caution in people with cardiovascular disease because of the risk of arrhythmias (abnormal heart beats). TCAs should not be used in people in the immediate recovery period following a myocardial infarction (heart attack) due to this risk. Some people with ID may not be able to give information on their medical history so this must be sought from other sources including carers, family and the general practitioner. A thorough physical examination will also be needed before starting TCAs.
- Due to the 'antimuscarinic' adverse effects (see adverse effects below), they should be used with caution in people with prostatic hypertrophy (enlarged prostate), chronic constipation, urinary retention, raised intra-ocular pressure and those at risk of angle-closure glaucoma.
- Older people are at increased risk of adverse effects and so low initial doses should be used with close monitoring.

The adverse effects of TCAs are:

- Effects on the heart such as arrhythmias (abnormal heart rhythm), heart block (abnormally low heart beat), tachycardia (fast heart rate) and postural hypotension (low blood pressure on standing), which could cause increase risk of falling.

- 'Antimuscarinic' adverse effects are caused by TCAs' action on the parasympathetic nervous system. They include dry mouth, blurred vision, constipation and urinary retention.

- Effects on the central nervous system, which include anxiety, dizziness, agitation, confusion, sleep problems, 'pins and needles', hallucinations, delusions and mania. TCAs can also increase the risk of seizures (again particularly relevant in people with epilepsy). Some TCAs cause drowsiness.

- Breast enlargement, galactorrhoea (production of milk from breasts), gynaecomastia (breast enlargement in males).

- Changes in appetite and weight.

- Hyponatraemia.

- Changes in blood sugar levels.

- Nausea and vomiting.

- Taste disturbance.

- May be fatal in overdose.

Investigations

Due to cardiovascular adverse effects a full physical examination and ECG including pulse and blood pressure should be conducted at baseline. Other investigations including blood sodium level and blood glucose should be carried out when indicated.

Monoamine oxidase inhibitors

Monoamine oxidase inhibitors (MAOIs) are another older class of antidepressants compared with SSRIs, which work by inhibiting the enzyme monoamine oxidase that breaks down the monoamine neurotransmitters serotonin and noradrenaline, thus increasing their levels in the brain. However, the action of MAOIs is not limited to the brain. They also act in the liver and gut. When a patient taking a MAOI eats food containing tyramine (a substance that can affect blood vessels), due to the action of the MAOI in the gut, it is not broken down. This leads to high levels of tyramine in the body, which can then can enter the blood stream and cause

Table 6.3: Summary of TCAs (Joint Formulary Committee, 2011)

TCA	Licensed dose	Main side effects	Main interactions
Amitritpyline	30–200mg a day.	As above. Causes sedation.	SSRIs (except citalopram) can increase blood levels. Also interacts with alcohol, MAOIs and antipsychotics.
Clomipramine	10–250mg a day.	As above.	As for amitriptyline.
Dosulepin	75–225mg a day.	As above.	As for amitriptyline.
Doxepin	10–300mg a day.	As above.	As for amitriptyline.
Imipramine	10–200mg a day.	As above. Less sedative.	As for amitriptyline.
Lofepramine	140–210mg a day.	As above. Less sedative. Constipation common.	As for amitriptyline.
Nortriptyline	30–150mg a day.	As above. Less sedative. Causes low blood pressure.	As for amitriptyline.
Trimipramine	30–300mg a day.	As above. More sedative.	Safer with MAOIs than other TCAs.

a 'hypertensive crisis'. This is a potentially very dangerous side effect of MAOIs (Joint Formulary Committee, 2011).

Examples of MAOIs include phenelzine, tranylcypromine and moclobemide. The following issues need to be considered when using MAOIs:

■ Due to the risk of a hypertensive crisis if a patient who is receiving an MOAI eats foods containing tyramine, certain foods need to be avoided. This includes mature cheese, pickled herring, broad bean pods and yeast extracts such as Marmite. Symptoms of a hypertensive crisis include significant hypertension (high blood pressure), tachycardia, arrhythmia and severe headaches. It can be life threatening. It may be difficult to explain this danger to a person with ID and careful monitoring of food is needed, which could be problematic.

- Certain drugs need to be avoided in people taking MAOIs. These include nasal decongestants, pethidine and levodopa. This is because the breakdown of these drugs is inhibited by MAOIs, which can cause an increase in their action on the sympathetic nervous system.

The adverse effects of MAOIs include:

- postural hypotension
- dizziness
- drowsiness
- headache
- problems sleeping
- dry mouth
- constipation
- blurred vision
- liver impairment
- reduced number of white blood cells in the blood.

Investigations

Table 6.4: MAOIs (Maudsley Prescribing Guides) (Taylor *et al*, 2007)			
MAOI	Licensed dose	Main adverse effects	Main interactions
Phenelzine	15mg, three or four times a day.	As above. Also weight gain.	Probably safest MAOI in antidepressant combinations. Tyramine interactions.
Tranylcypromine	10mg twice times a day.	Insomnia, nervousness and hypertensive crisis more common. Liver impairment less common.	As for phenelzine but reactions are more severe. Never use in combination with other antidepressants.
Moclobemide	150–600mg a day.	Sleep problems, nausea, agitation, confusion, high blood pressure.	Tyramine reactions rare and mild but possible with high doses.

Other antidepressants should not be started until two weeks after an MAOI has been stopped, and an MAOI should not be started until seven to 14 days after another antidepressant has been stopped. Due to the serious adverse effects of MAOIs, they are rarely used in people with ID.

Other antidepressant medications

There are several other antidepressants that do not fall into the categories of SSRIs, TCAs or MAOIs. These include mirtazapine, venlafaxine, agomelatine and duloxetine. The antidepressants in this class are often used before trying TCAs or MAOIs (NICE guide).

Mirtazapine: Mirtazapine increases levels of both serotonin and noradrenaline. The licensed dose is 15–45mg a day. Adverse effects include increased appetite, weight gain, drowsiness, dizziness, headache, peripheral oedma (swollen ankles/feet) and abnormalities in the full blood count.

Venlafaxine: Venlafaxine inhibits the uptake of serotonin and noradrenaline (an SNRI). The licensed dose is 75–225mg a day. Venlafaxine does not have the sedative and 'antimuscarinic' side effects of TCAs, but it can cause nausea, sleep problems, dizziness, sweating, sexual problems and headaches. In higher doses it has been associated with increased blood pressure, and blood pressure should be monitored and an ECG done at baseline. Venlafaxine commonly causes withdrawal symptoms, and so it should be stopped gradually.

Agomelatine: This is one of the newest licensed antidepressants. It works by increasing levels of serotonin and also altering melatonin levels. The licensed dose is 25–50mg a day. Adverse effects include nausea, diarrhoea, constipation, abdominal pain, liver impairment, headaches, dizziness, drowsiness, anxiety and sweating.

Duloxetine: Duloxetine inhibits the uptake of serotonin and noradrenaline. The licensed dose is 60–120mg a day. The main adverse effects are nausea, sleep problems, dizziness, dry mouth and constipation.

In certain patients, depression can be very difficult to treat. It may be necessary to 'augment' the antidepressant therapy by adding another medication. This should only be done in consultation with prescribing guidelines, including NICE guidelines. An antidepressant can be augmented with:

- lithium.
- an antipsychotic such as aripiprazole, olanzapine, quetiapine or risperidone.
- another antidepressant such as mirtazapine.

Case study: Miss X

A 19-year-old woman with mild ID presented with poor sleep and not finishing her meals. She was tearful and harming herself by hitting her arms and legs against large objects. A diagnosis of depression was made. The possible management plans were discussed with her, her family and her carers, and she was put on the waiting list for psychological therapy. She was also provided with an accessible leaflet about citalopram and helped to go through this during the appointment. She took this away with her to think about and at the next appointment decided to start on it. Her capacity to make this decision was assessed and it was felt that she was able to make it herself, and so she started on a low dose of 10mg to minimise any adverse effects. The dose of citalopram was increased to 20mg as she did not show any adverse effects. She continued to have regular reviews regarding her mental state and the prescription of citalopram. She has been advised that citalopram should ideally be continued until she has been well for at least six months.

Other treatments

Electroconvulsive therapy

Electroconvulsive therapy (ECT) involves passing an electric current through the brain to produce an epileptic fit. The idea for this treatment was developed at a time when there were no effective medications to treat mental health problems, but it was observed that people who had both epilepsy and depression seemed to feel better after having an epileptic fit. It is believed that in severe depression ECT increases the levels of the neurotransmitters in the brain. It should only be used for severe life-threatening depression (in patients who are not eating and drinking or for whom the risk of suicide is very high) or where other treatments have failed (Barnes, 2010). The seizure is induced by passing an electric current across the person's brain in a very controlled way using an ECT machine. An anaesthetic is given so the person is not conscious during the treatment, and a muscle relaxant is also administered so that the muscular spasms that are normally part of a seizure are reduced, therefore reducing the chance of an injury occurring. Short-term adverse effects include headache, aching muscles and the usual risks of general anaesthetics, while in the longer term there is a risk of problems with memory (Barnes, 2010).

Light therapy

Seasonal affective disorder (SAD) is a type of depression that starts in the autumn and carries on through the winter until spring, and it seems likely that a lack of daylight during this time of year is the cause. The symptoms are similar to non-seasonal depression, however in SAD, people are likely to eat and sleep more, which is the opposite of non-seasonal depression. Treatment can include the use of light therapy, which involves using a light-box that replicates the effects of sunlight but without the ultraviolet rays. If used for 30 minutes to an hour every day it can improve symptoms by making up for the lack of sunlight during these months (Eagles, 2010).

St John's wort

St John's wort is a plant that traditionally flowers on St John's day, 24th June, each year, and it has been suggested that it may be useful in treating low mood, anxiety and premenstrual stress by increasing the level of serotonin in the brain. It is available over the counter, however it can still have serious interactions with other medicines such as antidepressants, strong painkillers and the oral contraceptive pill. It can also reduce the effectiveness of some antiepileptic drugs, including digoxin and warfarin (Werneke, 2010).

Medications for the management of anxiety

As with depression, the NICE guidelines (NICE, 2011) suggest a 'stepped' approach to anxiety management. Medications are not advised as a first-line treatment in the management anxiety, which should instead take the form of low intensity psychological treatment. If this does not improve symptoms then the NICE guidelines recommend offering high intensity psychological treatment or drug therapy (NICE, 2011).

In terms of medication-based management, some SSRIs are recommended as the first line choice. When starting an SSRI, it should initially be prescribed at half the normal starting dose for the treatment of depression and gradually increased. This is because of the risk of increased anxiety when initiating treatment. A response is usually seen within six weeks.

Sertraline should be considered first as it is the most cost-effective SSRI, and this is recommended by NICE even though it is not yet licensed for this use. If this fails, a different SSRI (paroxetine, fluoxetine or escitalopram) or an SNRI (venlafaxine, for which an ECG monitoring is necessary) should be prescribed. If the person cannot tolerate SSRIs or SNRIs, pregabalin should be considered. Quetiapine (an antipsychotic medication) has also been seen to be effective in treating anxiety symptoms (Bandelow *et al*, 2008).

Pregabalin: This medication can also be used in the treatment of epilepsy and for people with nerve related pain. The licensed dose in generalised anxiety disorder is 150–600mg daily. Adverse effects include dry mouth, constipation, nausea and vomiting, flatulence, drowsiness, irritability, attention disturbance, disturbance in muscle control and movement, impaired memory, 'pins and needles' sensation, appetite changes, changes in sexual function and visual disturbances.

Risperidone: This is from a class of medication called antipsychotics. It is typically used to treat psychoses in people who have schizophrenia or mania in bipolar affective disorder. However, when given at low doses it has been shown to be very helpful in treating anxiety in people who have autistic spectrum disorder (Unwin & Deb, 2011). Side effects include weight gain, dizziness, postural hypotension, extra-pyramidal side effects (tremor, stiffness in limbs, slowed movements), increased blood sugar levels with a risk of developing diabetes, increased prolactin levels (which can cause breast enlargement), galactorrhoea and gynaecomastia. Investigations necessary at baseline are weight, height, blood pressure, ECG if at risk of heart disease, and blood tests include plasma glucose level and lipids. These baseline investigations should be monitored every three months for the first year of starting risperidone, and then yearly. If there are symptoms of raised prolactin levels then blood prolactin level should be checked.

Benzodiazepine medications should not be used in panic disorder. Furthermore, it should only be used for short-term treatment of two to four weeks in generalised anxiety disorder for a crisis because of the risk of developing a dependence if it is prescribed for longer than this.

Case study: Mr Z

A 29-year-old man with severe ID and autism displayed certain signs indicating that he was feeling anxious. These symptoms included holding his head upright, saying set phrases over and over again and grabbing people by their arms. Some triggers were identified that tended to increase his levels of anxiety. These triggers included unplanned changes in his routine, people offering too much choice, for example when deciding what to have for breakfast, people standing too close to him etc. It was felt that this anxiety was linked to his diagnosis of autism. Non-medication management plans were put in place including how to respond when he presented with the signs of anxiety and preparing him for any future changes. However, he continued to show anxiety despite behavioural management. It was felt that he did not have the capacity to give consent to his treatment. The multidisciplinary team therefore held a best interests meeting and decided to start him on risperidone. He had his weight checked, height measured and blood tests done. He was then started on a low dose of risperidone in the morning and evening, which seemed to help reduce his anxiety levels. He continues to have regular reviews for his medication.

Specific issues: treating depression and anxiety

There is limited research on the effectiveness of psychopharmacological treatments of depression and anxiety in people with ID. Most of the available evidence is anecdotal and based on case studies. However, it has been recognised that the management of depression and anxiety in this population is not principally different from that of the population without ID (Da Costa *et al*, 2011).

Specific reviews found that typical pharmacological agents were effective for depression in people with ID (Hurley, 2006), and since individuals with ID may be particularly susceptible to dysfunctions of the serotonin system, they may well benefit from the use of SSRIs (Racusin *et al*, 1999). Case reports have also demonstrated that fluoxetine is effective in the treatment of depression and self-injurious behaviour (Sovner *et al*, 1993). A study looking at the use of citalopram for depression in people with ID concluded that it was well tolerated, safe and effective (Verhoeven *et al*, 2001).

Reviews have shown that the use of ECT in people with ID is even rarer than for the general population, however they all report that its use is safe and effective (Kessler, 2004; Van Warade *et al*, 2001). Case reports have demonstrated that light therapy is useful in treating SAD in people with ID (Tsiouris & Iassid, 2007), while Altabet *et al* (2002) demonstrated the effective use of light therapy in three people with ID who had non-seasonal depression and sleep cycle problems.

Conclusions

It is essential that people with ID are treated using an evidence based approach, and more research into the treatment of anxiety and depression in people with ID is therefore needed. It can be difficult to organise robust clinical trials in this population group due to the ethical issues it raises (Oliver-Africano *et al*, 2010), however this is a barrier that can be overcome. Prescribers should follow the current available guidelines (NICE, 2009, 2011; Banks *et al*, 2007; Deb *et al*, 2009; Unwin & Deb, 2010), and use these in conjunction with their clinical expertise and judgement. A person's capacity to make a decision to consent to any medication prescribed should be assessed at the outset and the use of accessible information to support this should be used (Unwin & Deb, 2006). These guides advise that a thorough assessment should be carried out before a medication is prescribed. Before initiating medication, a formulation should be documented including the assessment and a rationale for the use of medication. Non-medication based management of problem behaviours should always be considered, and should be used either instead of, or along with, medication when necessary.

People with ID, their carers and the multidisciplinary team should be fully involved in the decision-making process from the outset (Hall & Deb, 2008). The time, methods and personnel to conduct the follow-up assessment should also be recorded at the outset. Both the impact of the intervention on the person's mental health and the adverse events should be assessed as objectively as possible, if necessary using validated instruments. At each follow-up, the original formulation should be reassessed, and non-medication based interventions should be considered along with the possibility of withdrawing medication.

Psychotropic medication, if needed, should be given in as small a dose as possible for as short a time as necessary. If medication is withdrawn, a relapse plan should be in place and the possibility of withdrawal symptoms in the form of problem behaviours should be considered before taking a decision to reinstate any such medication.

Ultimately, the aim of any management should be to reduce symptoms and to improve the quality of life of the patient.

Summary

- National guidelines should be followed when prescribing medication and used in conjunction with clinical expertise and judgement.
- Certain modifications may be needed when prescribing for people with ID.
- Capacity to consent must always be assessed when prescribing medication.
- More research into the management of depression and anxiety in people with ID is needed.

References

Altabet S, Neumann J & Watson-Johnston S (2002) Light therapy as a treatment of sleep cycle problems and depression. *Mental Health Aspects of Developmental Disabilities* **5** (1) 1–6.

Bandelow B, Zohar J, Hollander E, Kasper S, Möller H, Allgulander C, Ayuso-Gutierrez J, Baldwin D, Buenvicius, Cassano G, Fineberg N, Gabriels L, Hindmarch I, Kaiya H, Klein D, Lader M, Lecrubier Y, Lépine J, Liebowitz M, Lopez-Ibor J, Marazziti D, Miguel E, Oh K, Preter M, Rupprecht R, Sato M, Starcevic V, Stein D, van Ameringen M, Vega J & WFSBP Task Force for treatment guidelines for anxiety, obsessive-compulsive, post-traumatic stress disorders (2008) World Federation of Societies of Biological Psychiatry (WFSBP) guidelines for the pharmacological treatment of anxiety, obsessive-compulsive disorder: first revision. *The World Journal of Biological Psychiatry* **9** (4) 248–312.

Banks R, Bush A, Baker P, Bradshaw J, Carpenter P, Deb S, Joyce T, Mansell J & Xenitidis K (Eds) (2007) *Challenging Behaviour: A unified approach*. London: The Royal College of Psychiatrists, The British Psychological Society and The Royal College of Speech and Language Therapists.

Barnes R (2010) *Information on ECT*. London: Royal College of Psychiatrists.

Berney T & Deb S (2012) Epilepsy and learning disability. In: S Shorvon, R Guerrini, M Cook and S Lhatoo (Eds) *Epilepsy and Epileptic Seizures: Oxford Textbook in Clinical Neurology*. Oxford: Oxford University Press (in press).

Bhaumik S & Branford D (Eds) (2008) *The Frith Prescribing Guidelines for Adults with Intellectual Disability*. Aberdeen: Healthcomm UK Ltd.

Da Costa E, Koyee P, Bodgan N & Qassem T (2011) An audit of the management of depression in a community population with intellectual disabilities in accordance with NICE guidelines. *The British Journal of Developmental Disabilities* **57** (113) 147–157.

Deb S (2007) Epilepsy in people with mental retardation. In: J Jacobson and J Mulick (Eds) *Handbook of Mental Retardation and Developmental Disabilities* (pp81–96). New York: Kluwer Academic Publishers.

Deb S, Clarke D & Unwin G (2006) *Using Medication to Manage Behaviour Problems Among Adults with a Learning Disability.* London: University of Birmingham, MENCAP, The Royal College of Psychiatrists.

Deb S, Kwok H, Bertelli M, Salvador-Carulla L, Bradley E, Torr J & Barnhill J (2009) International guide to prescribing psychotropic medication for the management of problem behaviours in adults with intellectual disabilities. *World Psychiatry* **8** (3) 181–186.

Eagles J (2010) *Seasonal Affective Disorder (SAD).* London: Royal College of Psychiatrists.

Gelder M, Harrison P & Cowen P (Eds) (2006) *Shorter Oxford Textbook of Psychiatry.* Oxford: Oxford University Press.

Hall S & Deb S (2008) A qualitative study on the knowledge and views that people with learning disabilities and their carers have of psychotropic medication prescribed for behaviour problems. *Advances in Mental Health and Learning Disabilities* **2** (1) 29–37.

Hurley A (2006) Mood disorders in intellectual disability. *Current Opinion in Psychiatry* **19** (5) 465–469.

Joint Formulary Committee (2011) *British National Formulary No 61.* London: Pharmaceutical Press.

Kessler R (2004) Electroconvulsive therapy for affective disorders in persons with mental retardation. *Psychiatric Quarterly* **75** (1) 99–104.

NICE (2009) *Depression: The treatment and management of depression in adults.* London: NICE.

NICE (2011) *Generalised Anxiety Disorder and Panic Disorder (With or Without Agoraphobia) in Adults: Management in primary, secondary and community care.* London: NICE.

Oliver-Africano P, Dickens S, Ahmed Z, Bouras N, Cooray S, Deb S, Knapp M, Hare M, Meade M, Reece B, Bhaumik S, Harley D, Paichaud J, Regan A, Thomas D, Keratela S, Rao B, Dzendrowskyj T, Lenôtre L, Watson J & Tyrer P (2010) Overcoming the barriers experienced in conducting a medication trial in adults with aggressive challenging behaviour and intellectual disabilities. *Journal of Intellectual Disability Research* **54** (1) 17–25.

Racusin R, Kovner-Kline K & King B (1999) Selective serotonin reuptake inhibitors in intellectual disability. *Mental Retardation and Developmental Disabilities Research Reviews* **5** (4) 264–269.

Sovner R, Fox C, Lowry MJ & Lowry MA (1993) Fluoxetine treatment of depression and associated self-injury in two adults with mental retardation. *Journal of Intellectual Disability Research* **37** (3) 301–311.

Taylor D, Paton C & Kerwin R (2007) *The Maudsley Prescribing Guidelines* (9th edition). London: Informa Healthcare.

Tsiouris J & Iassid F (2007) Light therapy for seasonal depression in persons with intellectual disability: literature review and four case series. *Mental Health Aspects of Developmental Disabilities* **10** (4) 137–144.

Unwin G & Deb S (2006) *Your Guide to Taking Medication for Behaviour Problems: Easy read.* London: Mencap.

Unwin G & Deb S (2010) The use of medication to manage problem behaviours in adults with a learning disability: a national guideline. *Advances in Mental Health in Intellectual Disabilities* **4** (3) 4–11.

Unwin G & Deb S (2011) Efficacy of atypical antipsychotic medication in the management of behaviour problems in children with intellectual disabilities and borderline intelligence: a systematic review. *Research in Developmental Disabilities* **32** (6) 2121–2133.

Van Waarde J, Stolker J & Van der Mast R (2001) ECT in mental retardation: a review. *The Journal of ECT* **17** (4) 236–243.

Verhoeven W, Veendrik-Meekes M, Jacobs G, Van den Berg Y & Tuinier S (2001) Citalopram in mentally retarded patients with depression: a long-term clinical investigation. *European Psychiatry* **16** (2) 104–108.

Werneke U (2010) *Complementary and Alternative Medicines 1*. London: Royal College of Psychiatrists.

Chapter 7

Cognitive therapy

Dave Dagnan

Overview

This chapter provides an overview of a cognitive behavioural understanding of depression and anxiety, and describes associated interventions. The chapter begins by identifying the approaches to cognitive therapy that have been applied to people with ID and will then discuss issues in therapy processes, assessment and interventions, as well as presenting case study examples to illustrate these. Finally, the chapter considers some issues in making cognitive therapies more widely available to people with ID.

Learning objectives

■ To understand the basic theory and background of cognitive therapy for treating depression and anxiety in people with ID.

■ To understand how cognitive therapy interventions for depression and anxiety that are suitable for people with ID may be carried out.

■ To reflect upon detailed case studies describing the application of these approaches to people with ID.

Introduction

It is actually quite hard to identify a clear definition of cognitive therapy, and in practice most cognitive therapy integrates behavioural interventions alongside cognitive interventions. Cognitive therapy assumes that if a person is presenting with anxiety or depression, it is likely that their interpretation of the world or the skills they use to interpret the world are playing a part in this distress. Cognitive therapists therefore engage the client in examining and changing their interpretation of the world around them, or help them to acquire new cognitive skills in the expectation that this will alleviate distress.

The literature on cognitive therapy identifies two distinct approaches to the role of cognition in psychological and emotional distress. Dagnan & Chadwick (1997) describe these approaches as associated with either 'cognitive deficit' or 'cognitive distortion'.

Cognitive deficit approaches identify that psychological and emotional distress may be associated with the absence or lack of skill in cognitive processes. Thus, some interventions teach people thinking skills such as problem solving (Loumidis & Hill, 1997), self-regulation or self-instruction (Korotitsch & Nelson-Gray, 1999). Skill deficit approaches have been widely applied to emotional difficulties such as anxiety disorders and anger management problems.

Cognitive distortion approaches, on the other hand, assume that people's emotions and behaviour are strongly related to the interpretations they make of their world. When these interpretations are unhelpful to the person and prevent them from achieving a good quality of life then cognitive therapy, based on the distortion approach, offers methods to explore and re-examine the beliefs that are unhelpful and arrive at a view of the world that is more helpful to the individual. Approaches based on helping people to examine their beliefs have been applied to a wide range of emotional and behavioural problems (Kroese *et al*, 1997)

There are now a number of reviews of cognitive therapy's effectiveness with people with ID (Sturmey, 2004), and the general conclusion of these reviews is that, although there is a growing clinical evidence base, there is a notable absence of good quality outcome studies and controlled trials. Although not the focus of this paper, the majority of controlled trials for cognitive therapy for people with ID relate to anger management. However, there are now accounts of trials for people with ID in depression using relatively brief interventions delivered by non-specialist therapists (McGillivray *et al*, 2008).

Theoretical developments

Recent models within a cognitive framework have begun to provide perspectives that take into account the social context of people with ID. For example, in one review on depression in people with ID, Jahoda *et al*

(2006) suggest that continued exposure to low expectation, discrimination and devalued status may lead to cognitive experiences such as negative self-evaluation and low self-esteem. There is now a growing evidence base that identifies these as strongly associated with depression and anxiety (Dagnan & Sandhu, 1999). This work also identifies that cognitive therapy assumes that people have a reasonable degree of autonomy in their lives, and that they can make changes to their situations that will enable them to practice new skills and behave according to new insights gained from therapy. However, Jahoda *et al* (2006) identify that people with ID often live in contexts where their autonomy is severely limited, and that there may therefore be a significant role for the therapist to play in enabling the client's context to change in order to support the new skills they are developing in therapy.

A similar contextualised approach to anxiety disorders is suggested by Dagnan and Jahoda (2006). They reviewed the literature that describes developmental susceptibility to anxiety disorders with a particular emphasis on social anxiety, and identify that many of the developmental themes that are known to be associated with anxiety disorders are more likely to be present in the lives of people with ID than in the lives of people without. They then go on to consider the need to adapt therapy for people with ID based upon their particular social experience. They identify that the 'mainstream' model of social phobia and social anxiety assumes that social anxiety is associated with an over-estimation by the individual of the degree to which their behaviour in social contexts is negatively evaluated by others. Interventions then challenge these beliefs by providing accurate feedback on the person's performance in such situations. Dagnan and Jahoda (2006) point out that this may not be a valid approach for people with ID, whose disabled status and appearance may objectively change the way in which people evaluate and interact with them.

Readiness for therapy, therapy relationship and motivation

When considering the application of therapy to people with ID, it is important to consider their experiences of therapy as there is considerable evidence that outcomes will be significantly affected by the way in which therapy is offered. For example, it is well established that positive expectations of therapy influence positive outcomes. However, many people with ID will enter therapy without previous experience or any clear view as to what therapy is for.

Kilbane and Jahoda (2011) discuss the need to develop a positive expectation of therapy early on in the therapy process, and they describe a scale that can be used to measure this. It is also well established that a strong therapeutic relationship is important for the outcome. However, developing a positive therapeutic alliance with people with ID presents some challenges. Bordin (1979) suggested that the therapeutic alliance consists of three components:

- shared tasks
- shared goals
- a core emotional bond.

Waddington (2002) reviewed features of the therapeutic relationship in cognitive therapy and identified that while some therapies see it as the medium through which change is bought about, cognitive therapy sees the relationship as socially reinforcing and thus the aspect of therapy that keeps people coming back, when the techniques are not yet working. Waddington also identified that good therapy and shared successes actually lead to the formation of strong therapeutic relationships, rather than working the other way round (as may often be assumed), with the strong relationship being formed before significant therapeutic achievement.

Thus, therapeutic relationships with people with ID can be strengthened through attention to the core therapeutic skills of reflection, summarising and other empathy-conveying processes such as positive facial expression and nodding. These will allow the client to understand and experience the 'bonding' element of the therapeutic relationship. The therapist should also emphasise the development of shared goals, by clearly identifying the problem that brings the client to therapy, the overall goals of therapy, and the short-term goals.

The structure and techniques of cognitive therapy lend themselves to shared goals, as it has a collaborative approach and uses clear goal-setting and monitoring techniques, such as homework reviews and agenda setting. Finally, the therapist should emphasise shared tasks by frequently identifying small achievements in therapy. The therapist might encourage the client with ID to celebrate small achievements such as completing the agenda, completing assessments, completing a role play and so on.

Assessment

Cognitive therapy presents a range of emotional, cognitive and intellectual challenges to the client. Dagnan *et al* (2009) describe the assessment of some of the core skills associated with cognitive therapy so that therapy can be adapted to the individual's needs. They suggest that it is important to:

- assess the person's receptive and expressive language abilities in order to determine the complexity of language that will be safe to use
- assess the person's ability to recognise emotion in themselves and others and their 'usual' emotional language
- assess the person's ability to understand how the events in their external world affect their internal emotions
- assess how well they are able to understand the idea of 'cognition', and whether they are aware of what they 'say to themselves' in different situations.

In assessing anxiety and depression in people with ID it is important to determine which words the client uses and which they are able to recognise to describe their emotional experience. Many people with ID have relatively limited expressive vocabularies in the area of emotion and so discussing the words the person has to describe emotions, understanding what they mean to the person, and noting them so that you use them consistently within therapy will be important. Similarly, in discussing the physiological experiences of anxiety and depression it will be important to identify a language that people are able to understand. Many people with ID, for example, also find it hard to describe their internal experiences, and the use of figurative language (eg 'butterflies in the stomach'), may help some people while causing confusion in others.

As in any clinical intervention, it is important to use standardised measures to determine outcome where possible. In the area of anxiety and depression there are a number of possible measures available. The literature has examples of scales developed specifically for people with ID that have been adapted from those used in mainstream services, and the use of scales from mainstream services in un-adapted formats (Dagnan & Lindsay, 2004).

Although it is impossible to review all scales suitable for establishing outcomes in cognitive therapy, there are a small number of self-report scales that should be mentioned. The Glasgow Anxiety Scale (Mindham

& Espie, 2003) and the Glasgow Depression Scale (Cuthill *et al*, 2003) are both self-report scales developed specifically for people with ID. They are relatively unique in that their psychometric properties include 'cut-offs' for clinical and non-clinical presentation. There are also self-report scales for underlying psychological experiences in depression and anxiety such as self-esteem and social comparison (Dagnan & Sandhu, 1999) that are well used in this area.

Intervention

Cognitive therapy for people with ID often requires careful adaptation to meet their needs, and there are a number of key areas in which therapy is typically adapted for this population (Whitehouse *et al*, 2006).

Cognitive therapy with people with ID is often less complex than when applied to people without ID. The aim should be to implement a smaller number of interventions well, rather than try to effect a wide ranging and complex intervention. The presentation of information should be broken into smaller 'chunks', and the therapist should consider shorter and, if possible, more frequent sessions. The anxiety intervention described below is based on a 90-minute session that is broken into two thirty-minute halves with a substantial break for coffee and relaxation in between. The example of a depression intervention (see p134) describes occasions when the client is seen for therapy twice in three days. Inevitably, the language used within therapy is simplified and the therapist should pay careful attention to the length and structure of their sentences. Further to the idea that a smaller number of things should be done well, it is also suggested that therapy with people with ID may require considerable repetition of concepts and repeated practice of new cognitive, emotional and social skills.

The therapy process with people with ID is often more active than when engaging in therapy with the general population. Flipcharts or whiteboards are very useful for developing a shared agenda or for drawing and describing events and concepts within therapy. The therapist should often use practical and active methods to help them understand the events that cause distress, such as role play, drawings or even photographs of places and people in the person's life, as these may make it easier for the person to describe their experience. At times it may be useful to take the person into the places where they experience difficulties to get a richer sense of the emotional and cognitive processes that they are experiencing. Any skills to be tried out outside of therapy or any simple homework tasks must also be practices within therapy.

Therapy may also be more directive with people with ID. Jahoda *et al* (2009a) report that cognitive therapists working with people with ID ask many more questions than they would with people without ID. It is important to note that Jahoda *et al* (2009a) found that the process of asking questions in therapy did not necessarily mean that the collaborative nature of therapy was lost; they found that therapists were able to offer structure through question and agenda setting without controlling the content of the work, which was shown to predominantly come from the client. Structure and direction can be developed and maintained through breaking down activities into chucks, setting goals for each component and celebrating the small successes that make up the overall achievement of a goal or a task.

Finally, it is important to take the context of people with ID into account when engaging in cognitive therapy. Many people with ID live in supported environments or in their family home, and it can be very difficult for them to establish the autonomy needed in order to practice homework and new skills, and to start to respond to challenges in different and new ways. It may be necessary, or useful, to sensitively and carefully involve carers in the therapy process. This involvement can take a number of forms:

- The carer can be enlisted to ensure that opportunities to practice new skills are made available.
- A client may need help with their homework tasks.
- Carers may need education in understanding the nature of anxiety and depression.

Clearly the decision to involve carers should be made very carefully and the client's views should be respected, however it could potentially be a great benefit to the therapeutic process (Jahoda *et al*, 2009b).

Case Study: Anxiety

Mr A was a 25-year-old man with mild ID who lived with his mother and father in a small town. In the initial assessment interview, Mr A reported significant anxiety when alone in community settings, stating that he strongly believed that he would be attacked and that many of the young people he saw in his town were potential threats.

As far as could be ascertained, there were no simple trigger incidents in his history that had resulted in this anxiety. Instead, the formulation of his presentation was that he had heard other people in his family and social circles discussing the threats posed by young people in the community. Due to a pre-disposition towards rumination (his mother was able to identify rumination as a long-standing feature), he had focused on this issue and then, through a process of avoidance and secondary reinforcement, the anxiety and avoidance behaviour had become well established.

The anxiety caused a number of difficulties for him, however the two primary issues were that he rehearsed the anxieties repetitively when in the company of close friends and family and he had recently severely restricted his community activities. He did, however, continue to attend college courses three days each week and would spend time in close friends' houses at weekends.

Therapy was offered in 60–90 minute sessions, each of which was split into two with a 15–20 minute break that was spent making a cup of tea. The sessions included a core assessment of skills associated with cognitive therapy, which showed that Mr A had good understanding of the links between events in his environment and his emotional responses and some ability to provide mediating self-talk with respect to hypothetical events. He had a relatively poor emotional vocabulary, being unable to classify words related to anxiety, anger and sadness much above a chance level. The Glasgow Anxiety Scale (Mindham & Espie, 2003) was completed at the start and end of the intervention.

The intervention adopted a structured approach to teaching anxiety management skills. In the first intervention session, anxiety was normalised and it was identified that everyone gets anxious at times. The usual physiological response to anxiety was discussed and related to Mr A's own physiological experience. The therapist also introduced the idea of relaxation and encouraged Mr A to talk about the things he already did to manage his anxiety, and emphasised that relaxing our bodies helps us to feel less anxious.

continued >

The therapist then shared accessible materials that described anxiety and its experience. In the next session, the therapist went on to further develop Mr A's understanding of the physical and emotional signs of anxiety and identified his current and preferred relaxation and coping strategies. Mr A was also introduced to a simple progressive relaxation procedure that was practiced in the session, and was given a CD with relaxation instructions along with help to develop a plan for when he would practice the new techniques.

Next, the therapist discussed the link between behaviour, thoughts and feelings, and introduced role play as a method to explore how Mr A was currently managing anxiety provoking situations. He introduced simple self-instruction within the role play to demonstrate how Mr A might feel slightly differently if he said certain things to himself. At the end of each subsequent session, Mr A practiced progressive muscle relaxation techniques and any barriers to the practice of relaxation outside of sessions were discussed.

In the following session the therapist introduced a simple problem-solving structure to the role plays. This involved identifying the main problem (for example, 'I think I will be threatened by hoodies'), coming up with possible solutions (for example, plan to shout at them or to initially go out in the day time when young people are usually at school), selecting the best solution (the one that would not upset people but that would reduce his anxiety) and practicing this in role play and planning the next opportunity to put it into practice outside of the session. Further sessions then worked in the role play setting to generate key coping self-statements and to practice problem solving around two or three other areas that were causing anxiety.

Therapy for Mr A covered seven extended sessions. In the final two or three sessions, the therapist worked to consolidate the use of relaxation techniques, problem solving and positive self-statements. They worked collaboratively to build in self-rewarding statements and reviewed Mr A's understanding of anxiety and the management skills acquired in the sessions.

One area that worked particularly well was the use of relaxation techniques. The therapist discussed Mr A's current approaches to relaxation (listening to music, playing computer games) and identified the specific physiological features of his anxiety experience. Mr A then practiced a progressive muscle relaxation approach and found that he benefitted from this in the therapy session, and so he created a CD with a 10-minute muscle relation script, followed by 10 minutes of 'relaxing' music.

continued >

He was also able to use a simple problem solving approach to identify solutions to feeling overwhelmed in community settings, which included simple positive self-statements that were incompatible with his self-statements of threat from young people.

A simple cognitive restructuring approach was attempted with Mr A, however although he was able to engage in evidence-finding regarding the reality of the threat presented, this remained an 'intellectual' exercise and did not have any effect on his repetitive rumination.

Mr A and members of his family reported clear improvements in his presentation and his Glasgow Anxiety Scale score changed from 32 to 12, which is just within the range of scores not associated with clinical diagnoses of anxiety. Although at times he could still be very repetitive about his fears, he started to go out into the community with his close friend and was even able to go to a pub, a venue he had not been to without his parents for many years. In particular he found the relaxation CD useful and would spend time in his room listening to it before activities in the community if he felt his anxiety was in danger of preventing him engaging in activity. Further follow up offered a 'booster' to the skills acquired within therapy, and although he remained anxious and could easily return to repetitive thinking, he continued to engage in activity and showed signs of slow but consistent improvement.

Case Study: Depression

Mr B was a 38-year-old man with a mild ID who had depression. The intervention used included an activity and mood monitoring approach based on a simple behavioural activation model such as that described by Richards (2010). The intervention involved Mr B's carers in supporting agreed activities and in supporting them to develop a changed view of Mr B in the staffed home in which he lived. Mr B had experienced a number of significant life changes. His father had died two years before the referral and his mother had found supporting Mr B too stressful, and so 12 months ago he had moved into a small tenancy with two other men. The home had staff present for 24 hours each day; one member of staff in the house at night and several staff around during the day. Mr B had one-to-one support for activities for four hours each day. In the past four months Mr B had become increasingly withdrawn and was spending considerable amounts of time in his room refusing to engage in any activity outside of the house, and he was reducing his engagement in home maintenance.

continued >

He was occasionally tearful and at these times he would state that he didn't *'know what to do anymore'* and complain of stomach and head pains. He had undergone a number of physical tests and the primary care team were confident that there were no significant health issues underlying his change in behaviour.

Mr B was assessed using the Glasgow Depression Scale (Cuthill *et al*, 2003) on which he scored 28, indicating that he was in the depression range. Mr B was also seen by a psychiatrist, who did not consider him to be severely depressed and no clinician considered that he was a suicide risk. Thus, a psychological therapy was seen as an appropriate first intervention. Mr B was assessed as able to identify facial expression of emotion and as having a relatively rich emotional vocabulary identifying the words, 'upset', 'gloomy' and 'down' as describing his sad feelings. He was able to identify that he felt particularly sad when he thought about his father and that he felt that he just did not want to go out into the community with his support staff.

The initial phase of the intervention focused on educating Mr B as to the nature of depression, with particular emphasis on the link between depression and activity. Mr B was able to identify that in the past he had felt happier when he was doing more activities. With Mr B's agreement and collaboration, the key staff who worked one-to-one with him were also given some background in depression and the type of intervention that was being considered.

He was then helped to identify the activities that he used to enjoy taking part in, and he was also helped to identify the routine activities of daily living that he still was engaging in and those that were an important part of living in his house. He then worked on a hierarchy of activities to identify those that were most pleasurable and those that were hardest to do. He was able to use a 'hand width' analogue to describe how much he thought he would enjoy each activity and how hard he thought they would be. (A hand width analogue is simply using the distance between your hands to indicate how much you feel something.) Mr B and his therapist then agreed to a plan to start engaging in one activity. The activity chosen was the easiest and most pleasurable of those that had been identified. Although it was the most pleasurable that Mr B had identified, he did not expect to enjoy it very much and still expected it to be relatively effortful.

The carers were then included in the session and the process up to this point was reviewed. Mr B's prediction about the activity was noted and he and the staff agreed to make a note of how the activity went and how much they each enjoyed it. The first attempt to get this activity to take place did not work; Mr B was feeling particularly sad having just had a telephone conversation with his mother and could not be persuaded to leave the house.

continued >

The therapist was subsequently able to identify some simple steps that Mr B could use to prepare for the activity and these were shared with the staff. It was established that Mr B usually felt happier in the afternoons, and so the activity was re-planned for this time of day and on this occasion, with prompting by staff, he engaged in the activity. The therapist had arranged a review for the following day (ie. two days after the last session).

Diaries are typically hard for people with ID to use. To develop the mood and cognition monitoring within the activity scheduling, the therapist used the following approach. Having identified the first activity, a diary was constructed for Mr B that referred only to that situation, and which offered a graded symbolic presentation of happy through to sad faces, and a graded presentation of a scale using a single analogue line with anchors 'really easy' through to 'very hard'. With the support of staff, Mr B rated his emotions and expectations of how hard the activity would be at the start of the activity and then again after the activity.

Through a collaborative process with Mr B and his care staff, the hierarchy of activities identified by Mr B was reviewed, developed and worked through over 10 sessions. By the end of these sessions Mr B was engaging in four activities that had been introduced through the therapy, and was spontaneously engaging in activities in house on an ad hoc basis. Throughout this process Mr B had learned that engaging in activities was never as bad or hard as he was expecting and he and his staff had begun to use shorthand in sharing their learning from these experiences, telling each other 'it will be all right on the night' and 'I'll enjoy it once I'm there'. By the 10th session Mr B had a Glasgow Depression Scale score of 13, which is just on the cut-off considered to indicate a not-depressed score. Following the therapy sessions, Mr B and his staff were able to work on integrating activity planning into the routine of the house and continued developing activities for him.

As Mr B became more positive and engaged in his activities, the therapist was able to engage him in thinking about his father and moving into his new home. It is interesting and important to note that, by this time, Mr B's thoughts about these issues were no longer depressed but were appropriately sad and reflective upon his life changes. He could still be tearful when talking about his father, but could accept this sadness and was able to talk about how he missed him and remember the positive times they had together. It was evident that the engagement in activity had lifted his mood and sense of self-efficacy, and made it easier for him to reflect positively on his changed life circumstances.

Anxiety and Depression in People with Intellectual Disabilities   © Pavilion Publishing and Media Ltd 2012

The future of cognitive therapy with people with ID

There are two clear areas that will develop in the future regarding the use of cognitive therapy with people with ID. The first is the development of a more structured evidence base. At present, the literature on cognitive therapy for people with ID primarily deals with case studies, with the only random controlled trials being small scale and in the area of anger management. A number of research groups are working on trials for depression and anxiety, and these will result in a much clearer evidence base and imperative to use the approaches, and in clearer and more structured manuals and protocols for the delivery of cognitive interventions.

The second challenge for future development is to include people with ID as much as possible in mainstream services. Recent service developments in England, such as IAPT (Improving Access to Psychological Therapies), have opened cognitive therapy up to a much wider client group than previously benefitted from the intervention. We need to learn how we can support people with ID, and mainstream therapists need to be confident and competent enough to extend their skills to work with this population.

Summary

- There is a developing evidence base for the effective application of cognitive therapy for anxiety and depression with people with ID.

- The social context of the lives of people with ID has a substantial impact on their experience of anxiety and depression, and cognitive therapy can be adapted to take this into account.

- Cognitive therapy with people with ID should be adapted to meet their individual needs based on careful assessments of their core cognitive and emotional skills.

- The application of cognitive therapy to people with ID will continue to develop, and cognitive therapy will increasingly be offered to people with ID within mainstream mental health settings.

References

Bordin E (1979) The generalizability of the psychoanalytic concept of the working alliance. *Psychotherapy: Theory, Research & Practice* **16** (3) 252–260.

Cuthill F, Espie C & Cooper S (2003) Development and psychometric properties of the Glasgow Depression Scale for people with a learning disability: individual and carer supplement versions. *British Journal of Psychiatry* **182** 347–353.

Dagnan D & Chadwick P (1997). Cognitive behaviour therapy for people with learning disabilities: Assessment and intervention. In: B Kroese, D Dagnan and K Loumides (Eds) *Cognitive Behaviour Therapy for People with Learning Disabilities* (pp110–123). London: Routledge.

Dagnan D & Jahoda A (2006) Cognitive-behavioural intervention for people with intellectual disability and anxiety disorders. *Journal of Applied Research in Intellectual Disabilities* **19** (1) 91–97.

Dagnan D & Lindsay W (2004) Research issues in cognitive therapy. In: E Emerson, C Hatton, T Thompson and T Parmenter (Eds) *The International Handbook of Applied Research in Intellectual Disabilities* (pp517–530). Brighton: John Wiley & Sons.

Dagnan D, Mellor K & Jefferson C (2009) Assessment of cognitive therapy skills for people with learning disabilities. *Advances in Mental Health and Learning Disabilities* **3** (4) 25–30.

Dagnan D & Sandhu S (1999) Social comparison, self-esteem and depression in people with intellectual disability. *Journal of Intellectual Disability Research* **43** (5) 372–379.

Jahoda A, Dagnan D, Jarvie P & Kerr W (2006) Depression, social context and cognitive behavioural therapy for people who have intellectual disabilities. *Journal of Applied Research in Intellectual Disabilities* **19** (1) 81–89.

Jahoda A, Dagnan D, Kroese B, Pert C & Trower P (2009a) Cognitive behavioural therapy: from face to face interaction to a broader contextual understanding of change. *Journal of Intellectual Disability Research* **53** (9)

Jahoda A, Selkirk M, Trower P, Pert C, Kroese B, Dagnan D & Burford B (2009b) The balance of power in therapeutic interactions with individuals who have intellectual disabilities. *British Journal of Clinical Psychology* **48** (1) 63–77.

Kilbane A & Jahoda A (2011) Therapy Expectations: Preliminary exploration and measurement in adults with intellectual disabilities. *Journal of Applied Research in Intellectual Disabilities* **24** (6) 528–542.

Korotitsch W & Neslon-Gray R (1999) An overview of self-monitoring research in assessment and treatment. *Psychological Assessment* **11** (4) 415–425.

Kroese B, Dagnan D & Loumides K (Eds) (1997) *Cognitive Behaviour Therapy for People with Learning Disabilities.* London: Routledge.

Loumidis K & Hill A (1997) Social problem solving groups for adults with learning disabilities. In: B Kroese, D Dagnan and K Loumidis (Eds) *Cognitive Behaviour Therapy for People with Learning Disabilities*. London: Routledge.

McGillivray J, McCabe M & Kershaw M (2008) Depression in people with intellectual disability: an evaluation of a staff-administered treatment program. *Research in Developmental Disabilities* **29** (6) 524–536.

Mindham J & Espie C (2003) Glasgow Anxiety Scale for people with an intellectual disability (GAS-ID): development and psychometric properties of a new measure for use with people with mild intellectual disability. *Journal of Intellectual Disability Research* **47** (1) 22–30.

Richards D (2010) Behavioural Activation. In: J Bennet-Levy, D Ricahrds, P Farrand, H Chritensen, K Griffiths, D Kavanagh, B Klein, M Lau, A Proudfoot, L Ritterband, J White and C Williams (Eds) *Low Intensity CBT Interventions* (pp141–150). Oxford: Oxford University Press.

Sturmey P (2004) Cognitive therapy with people with intellectual disabilities: a selective review and critique. *Clinical Psychology & Psychotherapy* **11** (4) 222–232.

Waddington L (2002) The therapy relationship in cognitive therapy: a review. *Behavioural and Cognitive Psychotherapy* **30** 179–191.

Whitehouse R, Tudway J, Look R & Kroese B (2006) Adapting individual psychotherapy for adults with intellectual disabilities: a comparative review of the cognitive-behavioural and psychodynamic literature. *Journal of Applied Research in Intellectual Disabilities* **19** (1) 55–65.

Chapter 8

Solution focused brief therapy

E Veronica (Vicky) Bliss

Overview

This chapter provides a brief introduction to solution focused brief therapy (SFBT) and its application to people who have ID, specifically with reference to the common difficulties associated with anxiety and/or depression. It draws on the limited literature available, along with the author's clinical experience of using the approach with this population, and will discuss the principles, techniques and role of a solution focused therapist. The chapter then uses a fictional case study based on a mixture of real clients to illustrate the practical application of SFBT in a therapeutic setting.

Learning objectives

- People with ID have ideas about their preferred futures.
- People with ID already have many skills that they might be able to use to attain their preferred futures.
- The solution focused therapist's role is to learn the detail of where the person wants to get to as well as to notice and name existing skills that might help them to achieve their aims.

Introduction

We know from available literature (Hassiotis *et al*, 2011) that people with ID experience higher levels of anxiety and depression, among other difficulties, than their non-disabled counterparts, though the exact prevalence of these conditions is difficult to determine (eg. Smiley, 2005). We also know from various histories of therapeutic interventions that behaviour therapy was the preferred treatment for people with 'challenging behaviour' as they moved from institutions to homes in the community during the 1980s (eg. Stenfert-Kroese, 1998). Until relatively recently it was thought that challenging behaviour was a product only of the learning disability itself, rather than a possible manifestation of any mental ill-health (Smiley, 2005). More recently, psychotherapeutic options have expanded alongside studies of mental health difficulties, to include cognitive behaviour therapy, psychoanalysis and cognitive therapy (Willner, 2005), systemic working (Kaur & Scior, 2009) and behavioural therapy.

Discussions of psychotherapeutic approaches to anxiety and depression alongside other mental health difficulties often surround difficulties in assessing and diagnosing these conditions in people with ID (eg. Smiley, 2005; Hurley, 2008), and it is often necessary for people to have a good ability to express abstract concepts verbally, such as 'more than', 'less than', 'better' and 'worse'. It is also frequently the case that people with ID are required to learn and use the language of therapy, and be able to associate a feeling inside themselves with the 'correct' word to describe it to others.

Additionally, the usual requirement for the client to have language skills excludes those people who have ID but who are not verbal. Therapeutic approaches for this population usually involve working with carers, although intensive interaction provides a client-centred way of interacting with non-verbal individuals that can help in a therapeutic way (but see Firth (2006) for a review of this literature). We will talk more about intensive interaction and its similarity to SFBT later in this chapter when we meet our case study, Beth.

More recently, SFBT has been appearing in the literature as a potential approach for people with ID and/or their carers (Rhodes, 2000; Stoddart *et al*, 2001; Bliss, 2005; Smith, 2005; Lloyd & Dallos, 2008; Roeden *et al*, 2009). One noticeable difference between the literature regarding more traditional therapies and solution focused therapy is that SFBT is not dependent upon assessment or diagnostic activities for treatment to progress. In SFBT, the onus is on the therapist to learn and use the language of the client rather than the other way around, as can be the case with more problem-focused therapies.

However, in the same way that adaptations can be made to improve the accessibility of other therapies for this population, the literature for SFBT addresses possible adaptations to accommodate varying expressive and receptive language capacities and the environmental settings (often unusual by non-disabled standards) (Corcoran, 2002). We will discuss adaptations a little later in the chapter, after first exploring SFBT as an approach in a bit more depth.

What is SFBT?

SFBT is based on a set of principles that are consistent with social constructionism (O'Connell, 2005), that 'reality' is a concept that varies from person to person and there is no objective reality out there for us to know. Critically, this means that a solution focused therapist does not know what the client needs to do in order to fix their problem. This is very different to medical models of therapy, which rely on diagnoses and corresponding treatments. Reality is understood through the use of language between two or more people, thus the future is something that can be negotiated and created through the use of language (O'Connell, 2005).

In this sense, a solution focused therapist can only know how to help a patient by listening very carefully to what they want to be different in their lives. A solution focused therapist can also help by taking note of any existing strengths and competencies the person possesses that will help them make those changes. Finally, a solution focused therapist can listen to how the client will know that they are making these changes successfully and moving in the right direction.

So, in order to do solution focused work, all the therapist needs to know is:

- what the client wants to be different
- what resources the client already has that will help them reach their preferred future
- how they will know that they are moving in the right direction.

A careful reader will notice a conspicuous absence of a diagnosis, a problem, or a formulation of what's causing the problem in the above list. There are also no recommended treatments for various difficulties or problems within a solution focused context. When a solution focused therapist begins a conversation with a client, they have no idea of what changes, directions or activities to recommend for that person. Even when people are referred to a solution focused therapist for something such as anxiety or depression, the therapist will come to the sessions not knowing what it is that the client wants to change or how those changes might happen.

Instead, a solution focused therapist will come to sessions with an insatiable curiosity about what the client would like to be different as a result of the sessions, and will have expertise in asking questions to elicit and refine this information. There are a few techniques that a therapist might employ to gather the information they need, although these may or may not be helpful for people with ID or their carers. It is critical to good solution focused work that the therapist develops a skill in really listening to and clarifying the detail of what the person wants, as well as the details of how they will know they are moving in the right direction. This kind of 'extreme listening' (Bliss, 2010) is qualitatively different from simply paying attention, and requires the therapist to empty their head of assumptions and theories of change. It requires the therapist to respect and value what the person says and to believe that people with ID are competent and capable of change. Listening this closely is, in practice, exhausting (Bliss, 2010).

Before learning to use SFBT, I used to work from the evidenced-based assumption that thoughts were related to feelings and both of those were related to behaviours. I used to try to help the client make a change in one of those areas with the view that the other two areas would improve as a result. Doubtless this is effective for some people and is exactly the right thing to do in some cases. I know that I used to listen out for things that confirmed the assumptions I already held and I expected the client to need me to tell them how to get 'better' from whatever problem brought them to see me. I used to ask the client with ID what they wanted from therapy, and most likely I listened to confirm my thoughts about what they needed. I had not routinely considered asking clients the details of how they had already coped with difficulties in their lives. I rarely, if ever, started a session by asking 'What's been better?', thereby starting off each session with an assumption that change for the better was going to occur and indeed had already occurred.

For example, when using an SFBT approach, I asked one person how it came to be that she, raised in an institution since age of 10 and given the job of helping the 'low grades' within that institution every day, managed to develop a sense of humour. Where did her respect for the feelings of other people come from? How was it that she learned to be so tidy and so helpful to other people?

I spent two sessions with her while she patiently explained how she learned these things, and learning together how such a difficult life (she was about 60 when I saw her) turned her into such a lovely person instead of the raging maniac I might have become in similar circumstances. I've been genuinely mystified at people who are so debilitated by anxiety that they curl up in a ball when they get into my office. How did they even manage to get out of bed, get dressed, get into a car, survive the drive, wait in the waiting room and get themselves into my office? They are incredibly strong people with quite a few skills. Even if they are only doing what people tell them to do, I wonder how it is that they come to be so kind as to care what other people want? Do they always do what their carers tell them to do? And if so, what difference does that make to the carers and to them?

SFBT was developed by making a stack of case files representing individuals for whom 'standard' types of treatments did not work very well. For want of knowing what else to do, Steve de Shazer (co-founder of SFBT) and colleagues listened to clients very carefully and took seriously the details of what their clients said in terms of what was helping and what was not (Hoyt, 2001). It turned out that for many clients, moving forward involved changes that were not related to the referral problem, and that all clients had existing strengths and strategies that could be employed in helping them to get what they wanted.

Figure 8.1 illustrates the principles of SFBT, along with potential techniques to help the therapist and client reach a mutual understanding about the aims and small steps of the change process. It also illustrates the role of the solution focused therapist in using the tools (or other more effective tools if needed) to bring the principles to life.

Figure 8.1: Interlocking aspects of SFBT

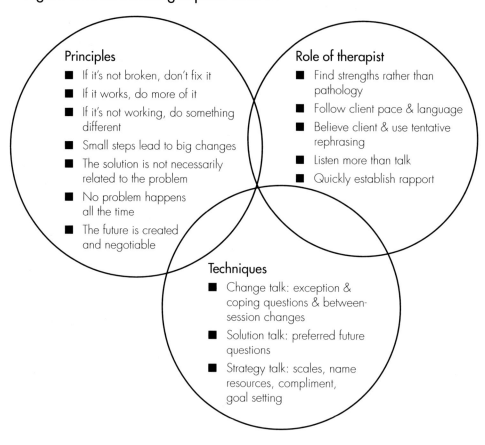

Principles

- If it's not broken, don't fix it
- If it works, do more of it
- If it's not working, do something different
- Small steps lead to big changes
- The solution is not necessarily related to the problem
- No problem happens all the time
- The future is created and negotiable

Role of therapist

- Find strengths rather than pathology
- Follow client pace & language
- Believe client & use tentative rephrasing
- Listen more than talk
- Quickly establish rapport

Techniques

- Change talk: exception & coping questions & between-session changes
- Solution talk: preferred future questions
- Strategy talk: scales, name resources, compliment, goal setting

Patrick and solution focused principles

To help illustrate the principles upon which SFBT is founded, we need to meet Patrick, a 59-year-old man with ID. Patrick looks like a man who has never lived in a house or eaten a good hearty meal. He chooses to wear clothes that do not fit him well and are only clean-ish, and he does not bother to comb his hair. He also has few teeth and likes to smoke cigarettes, even those that other people have smoked and thrown away. He is slightly built and moves very quickly in everything he does. One gets the sense that if he'd wanted to, Patrick could have had a rather lucrative career picking pockets.

Patrick was moved to an institutional setting when he was about 10 years old and has spent all of his life living very near to other people. For the last 10 years of his life he has lived in a flat with seven other people and full-time staff. His flat is one of several that have been made out of a large institutional ward on a campus where there are many such wards-cum-flats. On the campus there is also a small cafe, an art room, a working farm and a number of administrative offices. The site contains about 10 acres of arable land, buildings, landscaped gardens and farm animals. The local villages are about five miles away.

Patrick is a cheerful soul and likes very much to talk to people. He usually calls out across some distance when he sees someone he knows saying, *'Hey Vicky! Do you know me?'* with a big smile on his face. I had noticed Patrick out and about when I was on site and his skill at making people smile was truly remarkable. His questions were repetitive and his speech was difficult to understand if he ventured off familiar topics. He can smell a little to stand near, and yet at the same time it seems impossible not to smile in his presence.

Patrick was referred to me because he had stopped doing many things he ordinarily loved to do, such as helping in the garden, putting groceries away in the flat and wandering about talking to people. Normally a good eater, it seemed as though he was less interested in food and he often looked more tired during the day than usual. Patrick was referred by the people who worked with him, and so he himself was not necessarily a customer for change when we first met.

I was clear in my own mind before I met Patrick that my job was to listen to him, (using my eyes as well as ears because his language was not easy to understand) and to look out for his strengths, skills, future preferences and short term aims for our work together. I did not imagine that conversation with Patrick would be straightforward, so I had talked to the staff about the things he liked and came with a few pictures that I thought might help us have a conversation. It was also clear that here was a man with a lot of skills in 'getting by', entertaining himself, doing what he wanted to do, making sense of his world, managing his emotions, and interacting with other people.

It is important to add that before I listened to him, I had absolutely no idea if he wanted to do anything differently or what things might help him to reach his preferred future. This is different to a therapist coming to a session with a view of how behavioural change happens, as is the case with many other kinds of therapy. I really had no idea where our conversation would lead us to, or if it would be helpful to Patrick in any way.

When I met Patrick he chose to bring a favoured staff member along, and he eventually got me to understand that his preferred future was to stay in his current flat rather than move out into a community house. However, he realised that the plan for the overall service involved closing all the onsite buildings and moving people into smaller houses in the local community; a daunting prospect for many 59-year-olds, especially when the choice to move was not his. He was clear that he wasn't objecting to eating his meals, and said he simply didn't feel hungry. He found it hard to carry on with 'business as usual' because he didn't really know when he would be moving, where to, who his new staff would be and exactly what it would be like to move. He didn't even know who he would be living with or how to find these things out. I knew there was no option for Patrick to stay in his current flat and I knew that no one had advanced any specific plans about his move as yet so there were no answers to many of Patrick's questions.

I therefore wondered what things would help Patrick to cope with this uncertain future, and asked him how he would know that he was coping a little bit better the next time we met. I asked him about previous times when he'd managed change and asked what had helped him then. I listened as closely as I could to his ideas about what people around him might do to ease his worry. We discussed a need to eat well enough to be healthy and Patrick agreed that he might be better off eating more regularly like he used to do.

Let's return to the principles of SFBT and discuss how they applied to Patrick's situation.

Referring back to Figure 8.1, the first principle of SFBT tells us not to fix things that aren't broken. In Patrick's case, there were numerous behaviours that could be seen as antisocial. It would be understandable for therapists to want Patrick to pay more attention to personal hygiene, to wear more flattering clothes, to leave cigarette ends in the rubbish bin or on the ground, to slow down and think about what he's doing or saying, to stop asking repetitive questions or any of a number of other things.

In fact, several staff members wanted me to tackle these issues along with what was perceived as his 'depression', however I was prepared to listen to

Patrick in order to find out what it was, if anything, that he actually wanted to be different in his life. If something wasn't a problem to Patrick, then solution focused work with him probably would not address it. At the same time, if something was an issue for one of his staff, then solution work with that staff member would address it.

SFBT with staff groups is perfectly possible (Rhodes, 2000) and where there are groups, there are usually differing opinions as to preferred outcomes. In this case, it would have been possible to work in a solution focused way with the staff team around helping Patrick to improve his personal hygiene so long as they knew ways of doing this and had confidence that this was possible. If Patrick refused to participate in their plans to improve his hygiene, then the solution focused work would likely centre on helping the staff cope with his lack of hygiene as well as possible. It would be clear throughout the work, however, that poor hygiene is not Patrick's problem. It is within the preferred future of the staff team that Patrick's hygiene improves, not in Patrick's. Thus, for the purposes of individual work with Patrick, his hygiene is not broken, so we didn't assume it needed fixing.

The next principle in Figure 8.1 tells us that if something works, we should do more of it. This required me to talk to Patrick, and perhaps the staff, about times when Patrick had managed change before and whether or not there was any chance that he could be anxious about his move and at the same time be more like his old self with regard to eating, helping in the flat and going about his usual business. In terms of techniques of SFBT (also in Figure 8.1) this is considered 'change talk', where exceptions to the referral reason are explored to find out the details of what is already working. In Patrick's case, it seemed as though when certain staff were on duty, he would agree to get out and about more, and he could be encouraged to eat things throughout the day.

It was very important, therefore, to get to the details of how Patrick and the staff did this and to discover what difference it made to Patrick and the staff when he was more outgoing and amenable to food. It turned out that the staff who were having most success with Patrick were quietly spoken, calm and matter-of-fact about how they interacted with him. They told him what the plan for the day was, then set about getting on with the plan as though they expected no difficulties. They were light-hearted with Patrick, and if he didn't want to eat something they accepted this and moved on to the next thing, with a plan to re-present something to eat later on. Another thing staff noted was that Patrick loved helping other people, so if he knew something needed doing or a letter needed delivering, and the outcome of making someone else happy was made clear, Patrick was more likely to do the activity. We talked about how more of this could be done.

The third principle in Figure 8.1 tells us that if something isn't working we ought to stop doing it. It is such a simple concept that one wonders why we need to be told this, and at the same time it seems to be human nature to keep doing some things regardless of the outcome. Thinking about Patrick, the staff continued trying to coax him to eat at regular meal times and continued to suggest to him that he 'ought' to go out and 'do something'. Staff also frequently told Patrick to stop worrying about things that 'might' happen and just enjoy the present. They did their best to reassure him that no plans or changes would happen without him being involved and that nothing would happen if he didn't want it to, apart from having to make the overall move, of course.

These interventions had not improved things or changed the referral reason at all in the six months prior to Patrick and I meeting each other, and still the staff continued doing it because it seemed the 'right' thing to do. It is easy to keep doing what seems right, even in the face of evidence that it is not working. According to the principles of SFBT, we needn't keep doing anything that isn't working. It sounds simple and at the same time it can actually be quite difficult to do.

The fourth principle says that small steps lead to big changes. In Patrick's situation, remembering this was a relief to me because it meant I did not have to solve the huge situation that was causing him to worry. In fact, there was no immediate solution to his understandable worries because no specific plans had been made and the overall plan of having to move was not open to negotiation. I asked Patrick what small changes he would notice between our first meeting and the next time we met, that would tell him he was moving in the right direction ie. eating regularly and doing things that he was good at even though he remained worried at the same time. This is more 'change talk', as highlighted in Figure 8.1 under solution focused techniques. I asked the staff the same thing and encouraged them to notice when Patrick was more like himself and to point this out to him by saying something like, 'Even though you're worried, you still manage to make me smile!' This shows Patrick that we're listening to him, that we recognise he is worried and at the same time we're noticing the effort he is making to get back to 'business as usual'.

The fifth principle in Figure 8.1 states that the solution is not necessarily related to the problem. This surprised me when I was first learning about SFBT because I had been trained to root out problems, their frequency, duration, intensity, antecedents, consequences, maintaining reinforcers and triggers. I had been taught to hunt down the problems and all things related to it in forensic detail. Now I was being told I didn't need to know about the problems, and actually I could help people achieve their preferred future without ever talking about the problems. The language used to talk about problems is mainly historical, while the language of solution focused work is future oriented and contains implicit assumptions that change is inevitable, so whatever difficulty someone is having cannot stay the same forever.

It is also vital that the language of SFBT is matched to that of the client. In Patrick's case, I was a slow learner because he talked quickly and missed out some words all together. Patrick was very patient with me however, which was another skill I stored in my head in case it later came in handy in reaching his preferred future. Patrick was sensible enough to invite along a staff member who knew him well, who could act as an interpreter, and this helped me understand and match his language as best I could.

When Patrick and I did talk about the past, it was in the context of him recalling how he had managed upheavals before. I was keen to hear what things had and had not been helpful during any previous changes in case some of them could be used or avoided this time. I was careful to recognise the depth of Patrick's worry and at the same time recognise the depth of his strengths and resources, which allowed me to assume that he was going to cope with this upcoming change. Not coping was never mentioned as an option.

The next principle says that no problem happens all the time. We looked at the times when Patrick had gone about his business as usual even though he was worried. I asked staff for the details of when he had eaten well, when he had helped with chores, and when he had done the things he liked doing between the time he was referred and the time of our first appointment. I asked Patrick about times when he felt less worried or when he felt worried but it didn't bother him quite so much. These are difficult questions to answer and they are often unexpected questions to be asked during the course of psychological therapy. At the same time, they are worth spending time on because once people recognise there are already times when their preferred future is happening a little bit, they are already on the road to doing something differently.

The final principle states that the future is both created and negotiable. In keeping with a social constructionist base, solution focused work is centred on creating a person's preferred future through conversations. The more a person talks about what they want to be different, the more likely they are to notice when those things happen in their lives. For Patrick, I tried to use the word 'and' instead of the word 'but' when talking about the referral reasons and his preferred future. Just this little grammatical change sends the message that a person can be worried about something and go about life as usual at the same time, at least for some of the time. Thus came my question to Patrick regarding whether or not he could be both worried and manage to eat sensibly during the day. Could he be worried and carry on helping with the groceries, doing the garden or walking about the campus making people smile? The word 'and' allows two things to be true at the same time, whereas we so often negate the first part of a sentence by using the word 'but' in the middle.

Another linguistic manoeuvre is to use hopeful phrasing such as 'right now you are worried', because the implicit message here is that 'later you will not be'. It makes 'worried' a transient state that will not last forever.

Beth and non-verbal SFBT

Looking back at Figure 8.1, we can see that the techniques of SFBT are generally verbal, however many people with ID have limited language skills and therefore find it hard to carry on a conversation. This does not of course preclude them from having mental health difficulties, but it does exclude them from 'talking therapies'. Therapeutic work for non-verbal people is usually carried out with their carers, and there is at least one example of SFBT being used with carers in this way (Rhodes, 2000). For a solution focused therapist, the challenge is to find exceptions to difficulties by asking people who know the client well, but also using other senses, such as sight and touch, to gather information from the client. Noticing when the person makes a choice, for example, might be a clue towards learning a preferred future. As always, a guess at a preferred future is tentative and needs confirming by further watching and talking to carers. Exceptions and coping strategies might be noticed when activities are constructed in such a way as to maximise the chances of success, the details of which a therapist could get from carers. What follows is a brief example of working in this way.

Beth was a person with ID who was non-verbal, and yet at the same time she was able to teach me a great deal about what things were and were not important for her. She was also quite good at showing me what things she liked and did not like, often using an unequivocal slap of herself or me to make her point clearly. Her slapping, and occasional kicking, were very good instruments of communication and they heightened my motivation to get things right the first time by very carefully listening and watching her reactions. Fear of escalating her self-injury focused my mind quite sharply and it is always necessary to have a plan of fast intervention to diffuse self-injury when that is one means of communication used by a client. Self-injury is a reason to proceed carefully and thoughtfully, but it is sometimes used erroneously as a reason not to interact at all with a client.

Beth was a resident in a home for adults with autism and looked after by a skilled group of staff who very much wanted to keep her safe, meet her needs and help her do interesting things. At the same time, they felt challenged by her self-injury, by her limited vocabulary and by her impulsive behaviour that placed her at high risk in the community as well as in her home. When I met Beth, the staff voiced a preferred future that involved helping Beth to participate more fully in her own life, perhaps by making choices or by doing some of her own self-care. She spent most of her days in a specially made chair flicking magazines on her face, regurgitating and playing with saliva, rocking severely and screaming. The main contact she had with carers was verbal directions given from a distance because they worried that getting in her personal space would increase her self-injury or cause an injury to staff. I therefore asked the staff if they were confident they would be able to achieve their preferred future without entering her personal space, and we decided these two things were incompatible. This made it clear that the intervention would therefore involve finding a way to safely enter Beth's personal space.

Asking the carers for detailed information about all the times they could think of when Beth responded in unexpectedly positive ways yielded some information about her interests and their own skills in getting the best out of her. It turned out that Beth really seemed to like the feel of water, hand lotion, saliva, vomit and most other forms of liquid. She liked eye contact from carers some of the time and her rocking/slapping decreased when staff talked to her or laughed with her. She seemed to like the feel of soft or wet things on her face and hands and did not like it when these things were taken away.

With permission from Beth's guardian, I made a brief DVD of typical interactions with carers, then asked them to decide which kind of skill they thought Beth would most likely engage with as a first step. We guessed something with water might be in her preferred future, at least in the short term.

Using knowledge of what works from a behavioural perspective, I set up a situation where Beth and I would transfer three pegs from a soapy tub of water to another tub of water and then we'd ask Beth if she wanted to do more or to have a drink. We set up the tubs, double checked our fall back plan in case self-injury ensued, started the recording camera, and then I stepped into Beth's personal space and matched the 'language' of her rocking. I touched her hand and said, *'Hello Beth, I'm Vicky'* then stepped out of her personal space while matching her eye contact. She continued to look at me, so I continued to look at (and smile) at her. I repeated this several times, introducing a little information about our task each time. The frequency and timing of these little introductory episodes were governed by her reaction. I trusted, as one does with SFBT, in her knowledge of what would work for her and relied upon her telling me if she wanted me to back off or stop.

Having observed mainly interested and calm responses from Beth, I stepped again into her space and we put both our hands into the water. Having successfully carried out the activity I held her hands and said, *'That's three and we're done!'* She then raised her hand to slap her face and I intervened to shake her hand instead. I asked, *'Shall we do more or have a drink?'* She laughed and put our hands back into the water. We did the activity three more times, making quite a mess of water on the floor but laughing and rocking together for all the time. By the third time, she shouted out *'Three!'* when we finished, which startled me because I didn't know she could speak! This discovery led to staff working out how to encourage more speech along with encouraging participation in self-help skills.

All was not rosy with Beth, however, and the above description perhaps does not do justice to the complex nature of her presentation. As an example of SFBT, however, I hope Beth's case illustrates the principles of doing what works, small steps leading to big changes, solutions not necessarily being related to problems, no problem happening all the time and how new futures can be created and negotiated by following what the client says is and is not important. A solution focused approach in this case was informed by principles used in Intensive Interaction (Firth, 2006), which gives helpful insight into how to follow the non-verbal language of the client in a similar way to how a solution focused worker would use a client's verbal language.

Taking a cue from the client, a therapist can match non-verbal language such as eye contact, smiling, rocking, tapping, and even making noises to join with the client's preferred means of communication.

In terms of my role with Beth, I was not interested to find out antecedents or consequences of her behaviour (with the exception of self-injury as I had a responsibility to keep both Beth and myself safe). I was more interested in hearing stories of what things worked and in learning the details of what works from Beth's carers and from my observations of her. I used verbal language sparingly, I used her rocking to establish a rapport, and I kept a lookout for signs that she wanted me to stop whatever I was doing. My role as a worker was to honour whatever I could pick up about her means of communication.

Conclusion

SFBT is a good model with which to work with people who have their own unique way of looking at the world. I especially appreciate how it puts people with ID into the driving seat and gives them credit for having survived the traumas and dramas of their lives so far. Frequently, people with ID have survived difficult times and kept their willingness to help, their sense of humour, and some degree of patience with people who are trying to take them seriously. SFBT does not require that clients accept they have a 'problem', and as such is a good choice of approach for people who are referred by a third party. SFBT respects the client's own view of their preferred future, even when this is different from staff or 'others who know better'. It is a transparent approach that keeps the client at the centre of the work, because without them the therapist has no idea what to do. People with ID know when they are being listened to and when they are being taken seriously. This in itself is something that helps engagement and when combined with talking about the details of what the person has already accomplished, a good working relationship can be established.

Summary

- People with ID know when they are being listened to and taken seriously.
- SFBT is a realistic, viable option for therapeutic work with people who have ID, even if they are non-verbal.

- SFBT is truly client-centred, using the individual's own expertise to help themselves along with the therapist's expertise in asking useful questions to clarify what the person wants and how they might take a step towards getting there.

References

Bliss E (2005) Common factors, a solution focus and Sarah. *Journal of Systematic Therapies* **24** (4) 16–31.

Bliss E (2010) Extreme listening. In: T Nelson (Ed) *Doing Something Different*. London: Routledge.

Corcoran J (2002) Developmental adaptations of solution focused family therapy. *Brief Treatment and Crisis Intervention* **2** (4) 301–313.

Firth G (2006) Intensive interaction: a research review. *Mental Health and Learning Disabilities Research and Practice* **3** (1) 53–58.

Hassiotis A, Serfaty M, Azam K, Strydom A, Martin S, Parkes C, Blizard R & King M (2011) Cognitive behaviour therapy (CBT) for anxiety and depression in adults with mild intellectual disabilities (ID): a pilot randomised controlled trial. *Trials* **12** (95). Available at: http://www.trialsjournal.com/content/12/1/95 (accessed March 2012).

Hoyt M (2001) *Interviews With Brief Therapy Experts*. London: Routledge.

Hurley A (2008) Depression in adults with intellectual disability: symptoms and challenging behaviour. *Journal of Intellectual Disability Research* **52** (2) 905–916.

Kaur G & Scior K (2009) Systemic working in learning disability services: a UK wide survey. *British Journal of Learning Disabilities* **37** (3) 213–220.

Lloyd H & Dallos R (2008) First session solution focused brief therapy with families who have a child with severe intellectual disabilities: mothers' experiences and views. *Journal of Family Therapies* **30** (1) 5–28.

O'Connell B (2005) *Solution Focused Brief Therapy*. London: Sage.

Rhodes J (2000) Solution-focused consultation in a residential setting. *Clinical Psychology Forum* **141** 29–33.

Roeden J, Bannink F, Maaskant M & Curfs L (2009) Solution-focused brief therapy with persons with intellectual disabilities. *Journal of Policy and Practice in Intellectual Disabilities* **6** (4) 253–259.

Smiley E (2005) Epidemiology of mental health problems in adults with learning disability: an update. *Advances in Psychiatric Treatments* **11** 214–222.

Smith I (2005) Solution-focused brief therapy with people with learning disabilities: a case study. *British Journal of Learning Disabilities* **33** (3) 102–105.

Stenfert-Kroese B (1998) Cognitive behaviour therapy for people with learning disabilities: conceptual and contextual issues. In: B Kroese, D Dagnan & K Loumidis (Eds) *Cognitive-Behaviour Therapy for People with Learning Disabilities*. London: Brunner-Routledge.

Stoddart K, McDonnel J, Temple V & Mustata A (2001) Is brief better? A modified brief solution focused therapy approach for adults with a developmental delay. *Journal of Systematic Therapies* **20** (2) 24–40.

Willner P (2005) The effectiveness of psychotherapeutic interventions for people with learning disabilities: a critical overview. *Journal of Intellectual Disability Research* **49** (1) 73–85.

Chapter 9

Psychodynamic perspective

Nadja Alim

Overview

This chapter starts by contextualising anxiety and depressive disorders in people with ID from a developmental perspective, and then summarises the different schools of thought that have shaped psychodynamic therapy (PDT) practice as it is known in the UK today. Conceptualisations of anxiety and depression from within these different models will also be proposed. The chapter will then critically appraise the general lack of PDT treatment research, and will review one study involving the PDT of adults with ID and symptoms of anxiety and depression. It will then introduce a working model of PDT, exemplified through a case study, before drawing conclusions on the use of the PDT in everyday psychological practice with people with ID.

Learning objectives

- To gain an initial insight into the development of psychodynamic theories and their application in conceptualising the experiences and psychological worlds of people with ID and anxiety or depression.

- To contextualise their learning through the use of a structured PDT working model, which is illustrated through a case study.

- To conceptualise clinical presentations in people with ID from a psychodynamic perspective, taking into account past and present experiences that have shaped unconscious processes, which become apparent through defensive mechanisms and emotional vulnerabilities.

Introduction

It has long been noted that people with ID lack access to, or do not receive, adequate psychological and mental health services, although their need for such services has been proven to be greater than that of the general adult mental health population (Menolascino, 1965; Carlson, 1979; Sovner & Hurley, 1981; Reiss *et al,* 1982; Lund, 1985; Myers, 1986; Reed, 1997; Dodd & McGinnity, 2003). Public services generally promote the use of cognitive behaviour therapy (CBT) due to its increasing evidence-base and short-term application (Roth & Fonagy, 2006), while poorer study designs and a resulting lack of an evidence base for PDT weaken the argument for this approach. (For a review of the efficacy of CBT and PDT with clients without ID, see Leichsenring *et al,* 2006.) Nevertheless, a small number of clinical trials look promising, and conclude modest effects (Beail, 2003; Prout & Nowak-Drabik, 2003; Sturmey, 2004; Willner, 2005), while an assumption of the long-term nature and cost-ineffectiveness of PDT may be disputed (Beail *et al,* 2007). Beail *et al*'s study (2007) of the dose-effect relationship demonstrated the effectiveness of short-term PDT treatments as effective for people with ID.

Developmental work provides powerful evidence for the possible impact of early social experiences on thoughts and behaviour, such as frequent experiences of failure (Zigler *et al,* 2002), and in fact Zigler *et al* (2002) suggest that these early experiences shape the 'personality' of children with ID. They suggest that these children are:

- more likely to depend on a 'supportive adult'
- more likely to hold a sense of uneasiness about meeting new adults
- less optimistic about succeeding when faced with new challenges
- more likely to depend on others to help with problem-solving
- less likely to obtain satisfaction from addressing difficulties and finding solutions to them.

Moreover, Donovan and Spence (2000) argue that developmental factors that impact on mental health problems may include attachment styles, parental anxiety and parenting styles, child temperament (with an emphasis on behavioural inhibition) and traumatic life experiences. Warren *et al* (1997), for example, suggest that anxious/resistant attachment styles at 12 months predict a range of anxiety disorders at age 17 years, and it is proposed that attachment issues may be important in understanding the mental health of individuals with ID (Clegg & Sheard, 2002). It may be suggested that attachment patterns are similar in children with and without ID (Carlson *et al*, 2003). In fact, social anxiety in people with ID may arise from stigmatised identities, and be further perpetuated by a number of factors including emotional distance within families throughout the person's developmental period, low family sociability, family concerns about others' opinions, the use of shame as a disciplinary measure and overprotective parenting styles, for example during the period of transition from adolescence to young adulthood (Neal & Edelmann, 2003).

Figure 9.1: Illustration of the suggested impact of early social experiences on personality style, mental health and attachment patterns.

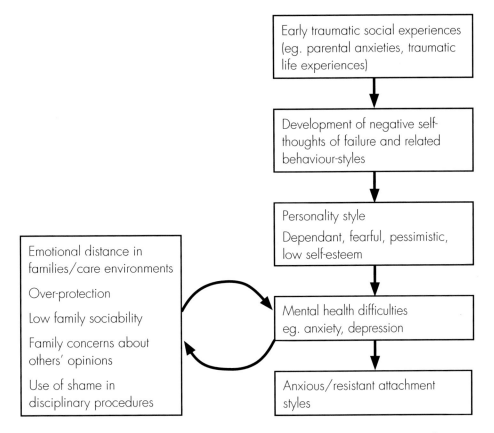

(Informed by Zigler *et al,* 2002; Donovan & Spence, 2000; Warren *et al,* 1997; Carlson *et al,* 2003; Clegg & Sheard, 2002; Neal & Edelmann, 2003.)

Applegate and Barol (1989) describe an approach to understanding infant-caregiver interactions that works as a model towards conceptualising psychological disturbances in people with ID. In line with object-relations schools of thoughts, they highlight the importance of early childhood experiences and suggest that parents usually repress worries and negative fantasies about their babies, and instead view their children more positively, as a potential affirmation of their own vitality and self-esteem. In this sense, the 'projective identification' process prepares the mother for becoming 'good enough' (Winnicott, 1970).

As a result, adequate holding and physical interactions foster the infant-caregiver relationship, thus promoting the child's self-regulation of both internally and externally generated anxiety. Here, parents foster the child's emotional regulation through holding, handling, touching and stimulating the child when in distress, leading to the child's awareness of internal as well as external worlds, and allowing them to appreciate the psychological sense of a separate identity. Through this capacity for 'indwelling in the soma' (Winnicott, 1965, p45), the infant's body-ego takes shape, defined by the skin as a limiting membrane (Applegate & Barol, 1989).

Furthermore, parental guilt for the child's ID and their inability to identify positive aspects of themselves in the infant may lead the parent to project their negative self-image on the child, and therefore compromise the experience of parenthood as a phase of normal adult development. In this sense, the secondary handicap of parenthood poses an intrinsic threat to the child's and parent's development and may complicate the dynamic between them. Here, due to the resulting reduced ability to appreciate the self as a separate identity, as is usually fostered through parental touch and nurturing, *'both a disturbance in primary narcissism and in the earliest steps towards a separate identity formation may result'* (McDonald, 1970, pp98–99). This may in turn lead to what Mannoni (1972) calls 'regression to the foetal stage'. A cycle of negative behaviours then follows that are met by parental frustration and neglect, leading to increases in what Winnicott termed 'unthinkable and unbearable anxiety' (Winnicott, 1970) and a compromise in the relationship between 'self' and 'other'.

Alternatively, and as suggested by Mannoni (1972), the child may feel that they need to live with the parent's fantasy that they are 'normal', hence themselves repressing acknowledgement of their ID. When the person subsequently fails to be 'normal' then this can result in difficulties with personality formation and low self-esteem, common antecedents to anxious and depressive disorders.

The theorists mentioned above conceptualise their thinking on the grounds of work with patients disabled by their emotional difficulties, rather than by ID leading to secondary emotional handicaps (Sinason, 1992). Work by Sinason (1992) and colleagues has pioneered the application of psychodynamic principles to practice with people with ID.

Relational psychological interventions for people with ID, such as PDT, may therefore be valuable in the treatment of anxiety and depression. These interventions use the therapeutic relationship to uncover unconscious or suppressed feelings with regards to early social relationships that are seen as central to the traumatic experience, and that lead to psychological difficulties. It is hoped that corrective emotional experiences (Alexander & French, 1946) within the therapist-patient relationship can override previous experiences and attachment patterns, thereby supporting psychological maturation and mental health.

The following Freudian, Adlerian and Kleinian schools of thought provide a background to PDT working models described later in this chapter. For a more in depth account, see Dryden (1996).

Freudian schools of thought

Freud (1923) believed that thoughts of guilt and shame, and aggressive and sexual impulses, are repressed due to societal rules forcing us to hide aspects of our sexuality/personality. This theory led to the conceptualisation of the mind containing three forces ('id', 'ego' and 'super-ego') that emerge progressively as the human mind develops. The id was understood as the biological core of motivation and the means of selfish satisfaction containing 'raw' sexual and aggressive impulses, ignorant of the external social world. In this conceptualisation, the id is innate and present from birth.

The ego, meanwhile, was understood to be the personality aspect responsible for co-ordinating internal and external reality, securing drive-satisfaction while maintaining safety. Simultaneously, the ego was also thought to somewhat repress the urges of the id when those urges threatened personal or societal danger. In terms of development, the ego was understood to gradually emerge during infancy.

As the human being becomes socialised, values and taboos of society become internalised resulting in the super-ego (Smith, 1996), which develops later still and further controls the urges of the id, acting as the arbiter of behaviour and ensuring that we conform to societal expectations. Freud (1923) further conceptualised psychological disturbance as a state of unmanageable conflict overloading the ego (Figure 9.2), against which the initial defence is repression within the unconscious. This repressed conflict, however, finds its expression in conscious awareness through, for instance, dreams, irrational actions and mood disorders.

Figure 9.2: Mind force-field conflict (Freud, 1923)

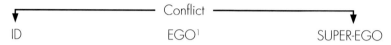

Modern neuroscience somewhat supports Freud's theories. Turner (2000) suggests that the human brain's evolution is three-fold, consisting of an initial primitive reptilian brain, a more developed mammalian emotional brain, and finally the neo-cortex, which is responsible for the higher functioning aspects of the human mind, such as language and conscious thought. According to Gerhardt (2004), this layer-perspective indicates mechanisms vital to processing and 'storing' memories/conceptualisations/ interpretations of experiences. Within therapy, psychological distress is suggested to be relieved through strengthening the ego by increasing awareness of previously stored material in the unconscious, which is believed to be at the core of the psychological disturbance. Freudian therapy attempts to help the patient to become more self-aware and able to cope with this self-awareness. Relief from psychological disturbance is therefore obtained through gaining a greater insight into oneself, facilitated by a suggestive and parent-like therapist, who aims to guide the patient through unconscious material.

Freud (1905) felt that psychoanalytic therapy would be most successful with individuals with a reasonable standard of education, suggesting that the outcome of psychoanalytic theory is positively correlated with the pre-treatment level of functioning (Bachrach & Leaf, 1978). However, outcome research has cast considerable doubt on this theory (Wallerstein, 1987). In line with a Freudian school of thought, one may conceptualise difficulties with anxiety and depression as a conflict of an underdeveloped ego with an overpowering super-ego. Here, difficulties with parental responsiveness and early attachments may lead to a lack of id-satisfaction in the early years

---

1. Resolves id-superego conflict through compromise; when conflicts are too powerful they become suppressed in the unconscious

and a parental over-emphasis on super-ego responses (eg. they place great importance on other people's opinions and convey a sense of shame in having a child with a ID, and so forth), which may lead to an imbalanced ego state. It is suggested that this results in a lack of emotional self-regulation, leading to the conceptualisation of the self as a failure and an over dependence on others for positive appraisal and emotional containment.

Moreover, possible unconscious processes in people with ID may be explained through Freud (1893), who suggested that memory of psychical trauma (such as the experience of disability) is a *'foreign body which, long after its entry, must continue to be regarded as an agent that is still at work'*.

Adlerian schools of thought

Adler's (1927) stance on individual therapy stressed the importance of observing the individual within their social context. According to Adler (1927), all individuals strive to develop a *gemeinschaftsgefühl* (feeling of social togetherness) during the early life stages. Here, the individual bases their learning about themselves and the world on observations of society/ family, leading to the development of perceptions. The person will attempt to behave in accordance with these perceptions, as these are believed to be the truth ('private logic' (Adler, 1927)). A person's behaviour therefore provokes the responses that are expected and that will hence contribute to a self-fulfilling prophecy.

Psychological health is accomplished through fulfilling the three life tasks of employment, social life and loving relationships (Adler, 1927). Psychological disturbance occurs when the individual feels inferior and not of equal standing among their peers. The individual then strives to deal with these feelings of insecurity by striving for personal superiority, and this discrepancy between feeling inferior and acting superior leads to the person being unable to accomplish the major life tasks because they are concerned only with preserving their own prestige rather than contributing to social situations. Private logic helps the person to explain their imperfection and inability to be truly superior, and avoids the need to attribute of self-blame (Adler, 1927). In psychologically healthy individuals, 'private logic' is replaced by common sense. Psychological disturbance is linked to early life traumas, where spoiled children will present with lack of self-belief in adulthood, criticised children become anxious adults and neglected children become discouraged adults (Adler, 1927; Clifford, 1996).

From an Adlerian viewpoint, emotional difficulties experienced by people with ID may be seen as indicative of the often unsuccessful striving for integration and societal acceptance through completion of the three life tasks. Failure to succeed due to societal restrictions, emotional malnourishment and cognitive and behavioural deficits may lead to feelings of inadequacy, failure and the development of symptoms of anxiety and depression.

Kleinian and object-relations schools of thought

Klein's work was largely dominated by her study of infant development. According to Klein (1952a), the baby develops an ego-sense the moment their vulnerability becomes obvious (eg. when fearing not being fed or nourished by the mother (Miller, 1983)). Furthermore, the baby is born with a love and a hate drive as needed for survival (Klein, 1952a). These innate feelings are in constant conflict, exacerbated by the infant's evolving life/world. To the infant, who is termed unable to distinguish between external and internal, self and surrounding, everything is objectified, even themselves. Furthermore, Klein (1952a) suggests that the conflicting feelings can be applied for one and the same object in rapid succession (hate for the lack of the motherly object, and love for the mother object when present). The infant is then said to engage in splitting the mother (and later, themselves) into 'good' and 'bad', as a need for survival, and then clinging only to the 'good' mother object and rejecting the 'bad' one (Klein, 1960; Cooper, 1996).

Furthermore, Klein (1952a) argues that the infant experiences intense greed, and becomes extremely demanding of the mother's care and attention, and anxious of being deprived of it. When the infant experiences the mother's distance (by growing older and needing to share the mother, for example, or by experiencing a mother who is psychologically traumatised or unavailable to the child), they will become envious. This envy eventually leads to their innate wish to destroy the loved object due to them withholding their love/nurture (Klein, 1952a). Exacerbated aggressive envy responses are understood as inhibiting good object relations and hence the capacity to love. If the situation continues, the infant and the mother are likely to develop depressive illness (Klein, 1952a; Cooper, 1996).

In this sense, Kleinian (1952b) concepts of the paranoid-schizoid and depressive positions are explained as follows:

- The infant is initially concerned with the threat to themselves (ie. paranoia concerning the realisation that the world is split into good and bad, as experienced through their relation to their mother).

- As the child's mind is said to split experiences more and more into these sub-sections of good and bad, the picture becomes schizoid and chaotic (paranoid-schizoid position).

- The infant's defences then help the organisation of good and bad, and unravel the chaos (Klein, 1952b).

- When these processes are stable and continual, the child moves into the depressive position, now seeing the threat to the external object and being able to conceptualise the objects around them (Klein, 1952b).

- The mother is now appreciated as a separate entity to the child, not simply as a source for good/bad responses.

- This provokes the separation anxiety, moving the anxiety from the paranoid to the depressive position, with the child experiencing guilt for their harmful responses towards the mother (Klein, 1952b). Furthermore, this stage is, according to Klein (1952b), also influenced by Oedipal envy and jealousy.

- Finally, the child's depression will slowly repair itself as they get used to being a separate entity and being independent (Miller, 1983).

Klein (1952b), Miller (1983) and Bowlby (1979) suggest that if the child experiences their fantasies as true ie. the mother as being bad or neglectful, or if they are prevented from splitting or projecting when experiencing qualitatively different object relations, they are prone to developing psychological ill-health such as depressive illness or anxiety disorders. This ill-health can be seen in the disabling of ego-formation in later life. The therapeutic relationship therefore aims to re-enact a healthy 'parental' attachment, leading to the patient's toleration of their situation and feelings by projecting them onto the therapist, thus allowing the patient to move into a committing, caring and understanding relationship (Cooper, 1996). Psychotherapy from a Kleinian perspective endeavours to help the patient move from the paranoid-schizoid to the depressive position (Cooper, 1996). From a Kleinian perspective, then, enduring symptoms of anxiety or depression may arise when an individual finds himself stuck at the paranoid-schizoid position.

The efficacy of PDT with people with ID

There are few PDT outcome studies within the field of ID. Difficulties with accurate diagnoses (see Einfeld & Aman, 1995) may hinder a more systematic approach to treatment of particular disorders and hence lead to a lack of outcome research. Hollins and Sinason (2000) suggest that people with ID can experience a range of post-traumatic stress symptoms. In adults and children, flashbacks, recurrent intrusive recollections, traumatic play, dreams and nightmares about a traumatic event, behavioural re-enactments and psychological as well as physiological responses to triggers of critical events are commonly associated with resulting disorders (Hollins & Sinason, 2000). It may therefore be suggested that people with low levels of cognitive functioning may react to trauma through disturbed behaviours that may be regarded as the psychological symptoms of depression or anxiety.

Nevertheless, difficulties with self-reporting and cognitive appraisal of traumatic events or psychological disturbances may prevent psychological diagnoses and treatment of people with ID, and compromise reviews of treatments and their effectiveness. Willner (2005) argues that the absence of randomised controlled trials in psychological treatment research with people with ID makes it impossible to distinguish which elements of therapy are responsible for therapeutic change.

Scotti *et al* (1991) remark on the relative absence of psychotherapeutic techniques in treating problem behaviours when reviewing the literature on treatment approaches. They further suggest that all studies involve single cases, with the majority utilising behaviour management approaches to treatment and the remainder applying medical treatments. Nevertheless, a number of papers have reviewed the process and, at times, the outcomes of PDT with people with ID (Willner, 2005).

Beail (1998; 2001) investigated the outcomes of PDT with offenders with ID, while Beail and Warden (1996) provided a course of PDT to people with problem behaviours (aggressive, sexually inappropriate, psychotic or bizarre) and concluded that PDT may produce promising, and at times long-term, outcomes in terms of low re-offending rates at six months and four years (Beail, 1998; 2001), or lowered levels of problem behaviours (Beail & Warden, 1996). However, treatment remained unclear, and Beail and Warden (1996) state that: '*The transference situation and counter-*

transference is used in therapy to understand the internal world of the client. Intervention mainly involves interpretation but in some cases containment issues are more significant...'. (p224).

Moreover, Beail (1998) suggests that: '*At a minimum, someone sat down with the participants each week and gave them individual attention, listened to them and focused on their feelings as well as their behaviour'.* This makes it difficult for studies to be replicated and PDT to become 'manualised' in a way necessary for outcome research.

Stoddart *et al* (2002) evaluated a bereavement group for people with ID in terms of whether their knowledge of bereavement and death increased, and whether there were decreases in reported depression and anxiety symptoms. Their study included 21 adults with ID, approximately half with a dual diagnosis and the other half only presenting with an ID. The authors assessed all clients against a variety of measures pre- and post-intervention (Kovacs, 1985; 1992; Meins, 1993; Parloff *et al,* 1954; Stoddard, 1996). All clients then attended a bereavement group intervention that appeared to focus on the therapeutic relationships and transference issues, and included practical exercises to support the management of grief.

Stoddart *et al* (2002) reported on five group goals.

1. To allow individuals to share their experiences and emotions surrounding their loss.
2. To provide participants with information regarding their grief and the mourning process.
3. To make participants aware that their reactions to the loss were not unique.
4. To help them move toward a new life for themselves without the deceased.
5. To assist the mourning process in an attempt to reduce the potential for unresolved or distorted grief.

They found that depression scores where significantly lower following the intervention. However, they also found that participants' understanding and knowledge of the bereavement process did not improve significantly. It was further suggested that while individuals with a dual diagnosis experienced a significant decrease in depressive symptoms, those with a single diagnosis did not. Generally, those with a dual diagnosis were reported to present with higher depression scores, while scores for anxiety were not significantly reduced.

The study may be criticised on various counts. First, relating outcomes to treatment becomes challenging due to lack of a 'no treatment' control group. Moreover, approximately half of the study participants did not present with anxiety disorders or depressive illness and so it may be difficult to compare these individuals' baseline functioning to those with mental health problems and include both types of participants in the same group. Although the authors did not clearly state their therapeutic approach of choice, it gives the impression of a psychoanalytic approach due to citing of Yalom (1985) as well as contemplation of transference issues in therapy. Additionally, none of the outcome measures used were standardised for adults with ID, while standardised measures for depression and anxiety exist for this client group. Overall, the outcomes of this study do not appear promising and do not promote the use of psychoanalytic/psychodynamic bereavement work. Furthermore, taking into account the shortcomings of the above study, its outcomes are questionable.

A major difficulty with PDT outcome research is the lack of treatment clarity preventing the replication of treatment. The following section aims to explore PDT working models that may help to conceptualise the treatment.

Working psychodynamically

Psychodynamic schools of thought suggest that at times of stress humans regress to more primitive or infantile ways of thinking, feeling and behaving (Jacobs, 2004). A person's reaction to stress is influenced by their experiences of early parental stress – stressful situations during childhood are internalised and, in this sense, objectified.

In suggesting a guided approach to treatment, Frankish (1989) adopts an understanding of the internal worlds and psychological development processes of people with ID based on Mahler *et al*'s (1975) theory of human development. Here, principles of maturation are adopted ranging from the earliest symbiotic relationship with the primary care giver to the final stage of psychological birth, which is separation-individuation. Within this model, the sub-stages of development are described as:

- differentiation, during which infants begin to recognise that there are parts of themselves that do not belong to the other, recognised by body exploration and looking
- practising, visible through the child beginning to put to the test its physically developing locomotive and vocalisation skills in particular, still with very close attachment to the primary care giver
- rapprochement, where the child experiments with increasing distance between itself and the primary care giver, but with regular and consistent reassurance, sometimes referred to as 'refuelling'
- individuation, where the child is able to separate from its primary carer with manageable or no anxiety and the sense of self as a separate being is established.

While the above model does not direct the therapeutic intervention, it does indicate the progression that a patient should take during a course of PDT. A different model, by Malan (1979), may support a more guided approach to therapeutic interventions, while adopting a predominantly Freudian and object-relational stance to therapy. Malan, following on from Menninger (1958), introduced stages of psychological development, aiming at conceptualising the personal growth experienced by patients of PDT. Conflict within the therapeutic/transferential relationship is believed to mirror current difficulties in the patient's life. These are suggested to stem from infantile/childhood conflicts/deficits. This therapeutic encounter is envisaged to lead to personal growth and ego-strengthening. Malan (1979) summarises PDT-processes by illustrating the triangles of conflict (ToC) and the triangle of the person (ToP) (see Figure 9.3). In essence, Malan's model provides an integrated summary of the Mahlerian, Kleinian and Freudian schools of thought.

Figure 9.3: The triangle of conflict and the person

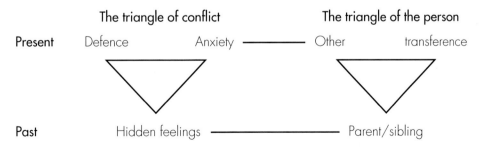

The ToP and ToC comprehensively summarise psychodynamic understandings of the psychological worlds of human beings and their development. Both triangles stand on apexes – one of hidden feelings (ToC) and the other of past relationships to parents/siblings (ToP). Hidden feelings (that is, unconscious thoughts and processes) and past relationships are regarded as underlying the remaining parts of the diagram, that is, the person's active experiences of anxieties that become apparent in the relationship to significant others in their present life and that are re-played in the transferential/therapeutic relationship. The anxieties are met through defences (eg. projection, introjection, aggressive reactions etc). In psychologically 'healthy' individuals, it is believed that a gradual understanding of one's own hidden feelings, impacting on relationships to others and leading to anxieties and defensive reactions, leads to a natural connection between the 'person' and their 'conflict', or, in other words, a connection between the ToP and the ToC.

According to Jacobs (2004), where relationships are disturbed (through traumatising events) the patient develops psychological illness leading to lower levels of conscious self-awareness. Here, connectivity between the above triangles is broken. In therapy, however, this connectivity is stimulated through the therapist raising awareness of patient–internal processes as exemplified through the transference/therapeutic relationship and as seen in relationships to other people in the patient's present life. The therapist utilises progressive interpretations enabling the patient to gain an insight into the relational processes and conflicts experienced in therapy. In this way, the patient's awareness of unconscious processes ('hidden feelings') increases and as a result PDT reaches beneath the defensive and anxious initial patient presentations to trace back feelings to the past usually as highlighted in family relations and acted out within therapy through the transference relationship. This process is illustrated in detail in the following Figures 9.4 to 9.12, each of which represents a different stage in therapy.

Malan-stage 1

Within Malan-stage 1, the patient completes the triangle of conflict, and indicates an understanding of the anxieties they experience in their relationships with other people in their present lives, which they attempt to cope with through defensive reactions. Furthermore, the patient's talk enables the therapist to understand the hidden feelings leading up to the patient's anxieties.

Figure 9.4

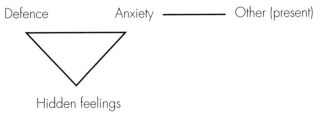

Malan-stage 2

Malan-stage 2 is described as the patient querying their relationship with the 'other' in the present through linking it to experienced anxieties and defensive mechanisms, and eventually linking the conflicts in the present to conflicts experienced in past relationships.

Figure 9.5

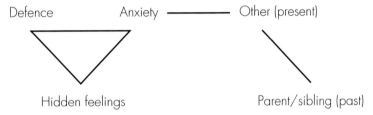

Malan-stage 3

Malan-stage 3 is acquired when the patient defends against their understanding of painful experiences with parents/siblings in the past as directly related to current difficulties. In other words, the patient briefly uncovers unconscious material/hidden feelings, before defending against their painful realisation. According to Malan (1979), the defence occurs by moving into the transference relationship and commenting on/relating to the therapist in a somewhat distraction-attempting way.

Figure 9.6

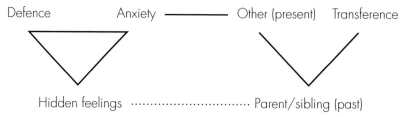

Malan-stage 4

Within Malan-stage 4, the patient initially relates their feelings towards the therapist to their experiences with 'the other', while the therapist aids the patient to reflect upon this relationship through the ToC. Malan-stage 4 is distinguishable from stage 3 by the therapist allowing the patient to move away from the painful realisation of hidden feelings as linked to past relationships to parents/siblings and move into the current relationship in the therapy-room. In order to get the patient to start contemplating the parent/sibling hidden feelings link, the therapist encourages the exploration of relational-patterns in the therapeutic relationship, as these are somewhat mirroring of the relationship to other people in the patient's life. The link between hidden feelings and anxieties as lived through the relationship to the other and as re-experienced in the relationship to the therapist now allows deeper contemplation of the therapist-patient relationship and the other-patient relationship.

Figure 9.7

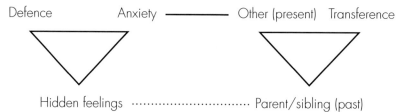

Malan-stage 5

Malan-stage 5 is signified by the patient's ability to contemplate past relationships to parents/siblings in relation to their now more deeply understood present (other/transference) relationships.

Figure 9.8

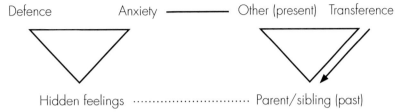

Malan-stage 6

Malan-stage 6 is signified by the introduction of the termination of the therapy. The patient is said to present with an increase in defences and anxieties as the end of therapy approaches.

Figure 9.9

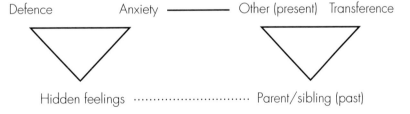

Malan-stage 7

Malan-stage 7 is signified by the patient acting out outside of therapy. The conflict arising outside of therapy is somewhat re-enacted within therapy and between therapist and patient, while it is suggested that the underlying source of conflict may be a feeling of abandonment as therapy is terminating. At this stage, however, the therapist can communicate the patient's feelings of abandonment in relation to the hidden feelings as triggered through past experiences and re-experienced through the relationship to the therapist. The patient is able to explore and endure the link to previously hidden/unconscious materials, signifying their understanding and that they are coming to terms with their conflicts.

Figure 9.10

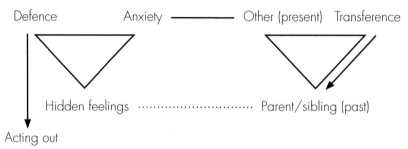

Malan-stage 8

Malan-stage 8 suggests that the patient again draws the link between their relationships with other people as linked to the transference relationship and as, in turn, directly connected to past relations (parent/siblings). This is in order to aid their understanding of the experienced 'rejection' by the therapist, as seen in the termination of the therapy.

Figure 9.11

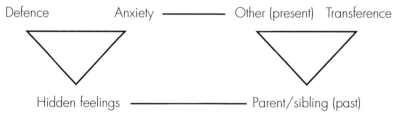

Malan-stage 9

Finally, Malan-stage 9 indicates the patient's completed awareness of the ToC and ToP, leading to heightened awareness and better conflict-resolution techniques.

Figure 9.12

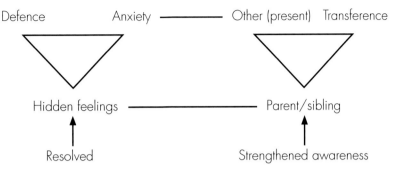

Initially, Malan (1979) explains therapy containment allowing the patient to regress and transmit their dependence onto the therapist. Experiencing the 'giving' of needed care will then lead to safety, which will enable the therapist to communicate to the patient that not all demands can be met (at the same time). The *'corrective emotional experience'* (Alexander & French, 1946) is therefore eventually understood as *'re-experiencing the old, unsettled conflict but with a new ending'*, and this is *'the secret of every penetrating therapeutic result'* (Alexander & French, 1946). In other words, the patient is enabled to reach the depressive position (Klein, 1975; Winnicott, 1958) and realise that ambivalent/opposing emotions can be directed towards the same person.

Case study: Jack

Jack is a 28-year-old white British man with cerebral palsy and a mild ID who lives in his own flat. He was born and brought up in the same area and his elderly mother and his three older siblings live nearby. Jack was referred to the community learning disability service due to low mood, self-neglect and lack of co-operation with services and supports.

Background history

Jack is the youngest of four siblings. His father worked as a taxi driver and his mother stayed at home looking after the children. Until nine months of age, Jack was said to have met his normal developmental milestones, and was crawling, able to sit up independently and make initial babble sounds with some intonation. He also showed interest in his environment and made good eye contact.

When he was nine months old, however, his mother left him sitting in a bath while she attended to one of the other children for a few minutes. When she returned, Jack had fallen into the bath with his head under the water and he was not breathing. An ambulance was called and Jack had to be resuscitated. Following this event, Jack's development was slow. He also stopped being able to sit up by himself and developed muscle spasms as well as stiff and inverted hands and feet, which led to an inability to develop both gross and fine motor skills such as walking and gripping. Jack developed some good language skills, although his developing speech was slurred and often difficult to understand. Jack was diagnosed with cerebral palsy at the age of two.

Jack's parents were traumatised by the accident and Jack's consequent disability. His mother blamed herself for the accident, as did his father who was very angry with his wife, although he also felt guilty himself. He began to distance himself more and more from Jack, while Jack's mother started drinking excessively and, although being very attached to Jack and highly anxious to ensure his well-being, she was often emotionally unavailable due to alcohol abuse.

When Jack was eight years old, his parents separated and neither Jack nor his siblings saw much of their father thereafter. Jack struggled in mainstream school, partly because of his language difficulties and his inability to make himself understood, and partly because he struggled to follow the school curriculum. Nevertheless, he learned basic reading and writing skills. He remembers making a couple of friends during his early school years and was said to have been a friendly and sociable child. At home, Jack struggled in his relationship to his older brother, Ryan, who would often exclude Jack from games or play tricks on him such as taking his wheelchair away and leaving him to lie on the floor for hours. Jack recalls a feeling of 'them and me' when remembering his childhood sibling relationships.

When Jack was 11, he started attending a school for children with special needs. Jack remembers feeling upset at leaving his old school and friends behind and did not feel like he fitted into the new school environment. Reports from this time suggest that Jack started withdrawing from playground activities and wanted to be left alone. He did not recall making any friends at the new school and did not want to be seen with other physically or intellectually disabled people in the community. He kept in touch with his friends from primary school and saw them occasionally.

When Jack was 15, he fell in love with a girl in a local coffee shop where he regularly met his friends. He was very shy and did not know how to approach the girl, so his friend asked her to join their table. Jack kept going back to the cafe and speaking with the girl, however after a few months the girl started going out with one of Jack's friends. Jack felt very upset and let down by his friend.

When Jack was 16, his brother Ryan, then 18, was arrested and sent to prison. When Jack, his siblings and his mother went to visit Ryan, Ryan became very upset and shouted abuse at Jack and said that it was his fault that their father had left. Jack became even more depressed and withdrawn following this event. He lost interest in food and became very thin and he was not keen to leave the house or meet his friends. He was eventually seen by his local child and adolescent mental health team and was prescribed a mood stabiliser. This helped Jack, lifted his mood and, while still being quite withdrawn, Jack went on to a vocational training course, learning hospitality skills.

When Jack was 19, one of his friends started working in a bowling alley and he helped Jack to get a paid job collecting glasses for the bar. Jack's mother didn't like him working there and would insist upon walking him to and from the alley, which could sometimes be in the early hours of the morning. Jack said that he hated his mother picking him up but that he could not convince her otherwise.

When he was 20, all of Jack's siblings had left home and he was keen to do the same. His mother was against this, however, and when Jack received assessments though social workers she would frequently talk over Jack and not give him a chance to speak. Jack voiced his frustration about this to a woman named Alice who he had become friends with at the bowling alley. Alice supported Jack to have a meeting with a social worker at her house and Jack was given a flat as well as direct payments to allow him to arrange for his own care support. Jack's mother was very upset by this and would often come to see Jack at his new flat to check whether he was managing.

Meanwhile, Jack and Alice had started dating, but he was not leaving enough money to spend on himself and arrange for support. Jack would often visit Alice in her flat and while he was keen to further a sexual relationship, he felt shy and ashamed to initiate this. Jack started to struggle to keep his flat in order and would often refuse to let his mother in, who would want to clean and tidy. He felt his mother's involvement in his life to be intrusive and struggled with her being critical of his relationship with Alice, often saying that she was just using him for his money.

Jack was also worried about their relationship – he was often unable to get hold of her for long periods of time, doubting her faithfulness and commitment to him. When Jack was 26, Alice told him that she had met someone else and ended their relationship. This devastated Jack and he became increasingly socially isolated.

When Jack was referred to the ID team, he was known to social services due to various complaints from neighbours as there was a strong smell coming from his flat, as well as concerns from his mother that Jack was not looking after himself, often not paying his bills resulting him being left without heating, hot water or a telephone. Jack would refuse to open the door to social workers and began appearing more and more dishevelled, withdrawn and emaciated.

He was offered four initial assessment sessions to aid the formulation of his case. Jack presented as withdrawn during the initial assessment. He very reluctantly presented his story and became tearful at several points, particularly when speaking about his brother in prison and his ex-girlfriend. Jack experienced his own tears as traumatic as his entire body would go into spasm and his sobbing would be uncontrollable. He later described his crying spells as 'break outs', linking them to uncontrollable volcanoes erupting. During this initial stage of therapy, Jack would want to leave whenever he started to cry.

Anxiety and Depression in People with Intellectual Disabilities   © Pavilion Publishing and Media Ltd 2012

Figure 9.13: Formulating Jack's case using the Malan-model

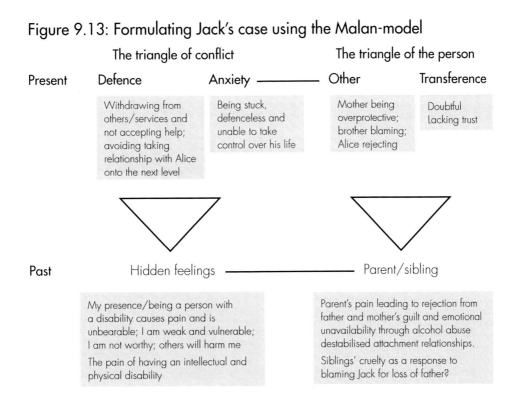

The triangle of conflict

The triangle of the person

Present

Defence — Anxiety ———— Other — Transference

Withdrawing from others/services and not accepting help; avoiding taking relationship with Alice onto the next level

Being stuck, defenceless and unable to take control over his life

Mother being overprotective; brother blaming; Alice rejecting

Doubtful Lacking trust

Past

Hidden feelings ———————— Parent/sibling

My presence/being a person with a disability causes pain and is unbearable; I am weak and vulnerable; I am not worthy; others will harm me

The pain of having an intellectual and physical disability

Parent's pain leading to rejection from father and mother's guilt and emotional unavailability through alcohol abuse destabilised attachment relationships.

Siblings' cruelty as a response to blaming Jack for loss of father?

The impact of the parental and sibling relationships on Jack's hidden feelings (past level)

As outlined above, Jack's case was formulated as follows. Jack's accident during infancy, which appears to have led to Jack developing cerebral palsy, was very traumatic for the family. His father's guilt and upset over Jack's disability led him to reject his son, communicating to him that he was unbearable as a person with a disability. His mother's overprotection and anxiety, as well as her alcohol abuse, furthered this belief and led Jack to see himself as weak and vulnerable. This was further exacerbated by his siblings, who ostracised and bullied him, leading to a potential hidden/unconscious feeling of 'being unworthy'.

This appears to have led to an insecure attachment to his primary care givers, and while longing for parental care and attention, this was widely unavailable. According to Klein (1952a), Jack may be stuck in the paranoid-schizoid position, envying that which creates the distance between himself and his emotionally unavailable parents, namely, his disability. This envy then fuels a depressive response, leading to Jack being trapped in an overprotective relationship with his mother. Mahler *et al*'s (1975) model may suggest that, due to insecurities around separation from primary care givers caused by a lack of emotional security with them, Jack has not yet reached a stage of separation-individuation.

Jack's anxieties and defensive reactions towards others and within the transferential relationship (present level)

Jack's pain of being a person with an intellectual and physical disability, buried in his unconscious, had to some extent been emphasised by others' over-protectiveness, and by their blaming and rejecting. High levels of anxiety were triggered by:

- feeling stuck (eg. with his mother's over-protectiveness and struggling to move on in his relationship with her)
- defenceless (eg. towards his brother's blaming)
- out of control (eg. feeling unable to develop his relationship with Alice, and when doubting her faithfulness).

In order to prevent these feelings from touching upon his hidden feelings, which were buried in his unconscious, Jack reacted defensively and withdrew from others. This could also be seen in the transferential relationship, where Jack left the therapy whenever he started to feel upset, unable to allow the therapist to provide emotional containment. In turn, this led to the therapist's transference response of also feeling incapacitated and stuck.

Following the assessment sessions, Jack was offered an initial 12 sessions of therapy.

The therapy as guided through the Malan-model

The first stage of therapy with Jack (Malan-stage 1) was marked by Jack's repeated disengagement due to his crying spells (defence). It became apparent that Jack was unable to allow the therapist to become emotionally close, and he therefore disengaged whenever his emotional world was being explored. Before the crying spells, Jack would often speak about Alice and Ryan (other) and how he felt he was rejected by them (anxiety). He would sympathise with them and say things like, '*Well, who would want to sleep with a spastic, anyway?*' when referring to his inability to further his relationship to Alice, which he saw at the core of its failure.

The relationship between Jack's anxieties and his hidden feelings became evident through comments such as this, and as therapy was progressing he was able to experience the therapist's continuity and acceptance of his feelings and actions (eg. by the therapist being there each week even if Jack would often leave the therapy prematurely). Through building this trust, the therapist was able to establish a relationship with Jack and understand his hidden feelings of 'unworthiness' as underlying his anxieties, which Jack was able to hear and contemplate.

Jack reached Malan-stage 2 in session 5, when he started speaking about Ryan and his sibling's cruelty towards him when they were children. He recalled one Christmas day, when his mother was highly intoxicated, spending the day in bed, while his siblings took away his wheelchair leaving him lying on the floor and used the chair to skid around the icy street outside their flat. Jack recalled painful memories of lying on the floor unable to move, with his mother not hearing and responding to his cries for help, while listening to his siblings laughing and enjoying their game outside of the house. Following this disclosure, Jack was able to say how ostracised and unwanted he had often felt and how he had wished to be included within groups of people without ID.

The therapist's responses to Jack were marked by empathy while highlighting the newly established link between Jack's present and past relationship experiences. Interpretative comments on Jack's accounts of present events and linking these to past experiences of rejection were accepted by Jack. He also began remaining in therapy for the entire session, even when starting to cry. He was able to tolerate the therapist's presence and appeared to experience this as emotionally containing.

Jack's transition into Malan-stage 3 could be seen when he delivered an account of his father leaving, having experienced repeated rejections from him. Jack described how his father would never take him out for a ride in the taxi and wondered whether 'he was embarrassed of me'. This realisation, that his presence was potentially unbearable, was then immediately defended against by Jack who asked the therapist whether she was married, pointing to a ring on her finger. The therapist was struck by his comment and became distracted by Jack's interest in her, with Jack almost appearing flirtatious. Following this session, the therapist was left feeling worried and it became apparent that Jack's question was likely to have been a result of his fear that his hidden feelings were being focused upon, and he therefore unconsciously distracted the therapist.

In the following session, the therapist attempted to move Jack onto Malan-stage 4 by speaking about Jack's question, and her interpreting that he may have been gauging how she fitted into the 'non-disabled' world, which he so longed to be part of. Further discussions of therapy then focused on Jack's fear of belonging to a disabled rather than a non-disabled community, and his fear that he would 'not fit into' the therapeutic relationship due to his feelings of inadequacy in front of a non-disabled and female therapist.

Jack then spoke about current experiences of rejection, such as his brother not speaking to him, his ex-girlfriend having left, and his fears over the infidelity of women. Jack was able to discuss his anxieties concerning the lack of control he felt he had over his life, his feelings of powerlessness and emasculation in his relationships with women, both in regard to his inability to have a sexual relationship with Alice and his struggle to maintain his independence from his mother. This was then related to his fears and fantasies for the therapeutic relationship. While there was a mutual acknowledgement of Jack's hidden feeling, the sessions' contents did not directly touch on this and the therapist did not yet make direct interpretations of Jack's unconscious processes.

Jack reached Malan-stage 5 following a cancelled session due to the therapist being unwell and unavailable. Jack and the therapist explored how this made Jack feel, and how his fears of inadequacy and being rejected had come true. Jack was then able to recognise a link between this feeling towards the therapist and his previous feelings towards his father. He explained how he was always 'living in the hope' that one day his father would take him out in the taxi, which would have represented the acceptance that Jack craved. Similarly, he was able to accept the therapist's interpretation of his hope to be part of the therapist's life and her accepting him into a non-disabled world. Jack was able to acknowledge that he felt enraged at this lack of acceptance and that he has similar feelings towards his father.

Anxiety and Depression in People with Intellectual Disabilities   © Pavilion Publishing and Media Ltd 2012

In session 12, Jack and the therapist reviewed their work together. As the therapy was funded by the NHS and there was pressure on the psychology service to avoid offering open-ended treatments, the therapist suggested another six sessions before ending the therapy. Jack agreed, but then did not attend the following two therapy sessions without cancelling, which led the therapist to conclude that Jack had entered Malan-stage 6, whereby he was reverting to his old defence of disengaging due to feelings of rejection.

Just before the next therapy session, the therapist received a telephone call from Jack's social worker who explained that Jack's flat had been flooded after he ran himself a bath and not turned off the taps, and he was now housed in a respite service with other people with ID until a new flat had been found.

In this new accommodation, Jack had been observed to be verbally aggressive towards the other residents. When Jack next attended the therapy, he appeared aroused and angry. When the therapist addressed his non-attendance, he told her that he had more important things to worry about and that he was now housed with 'spastics', and wanted her to 'get him out of there'. The therapist responded by acknowledging that Jack was in a bad place and that he wanted to escape. Jack then verbally abused the therapist saying that she was 'no good' and that she has 'been useless'. The therapist was able to sensitively interpret that it was really Jack who felt like that and suggested that he may be struggling with the termination of the therapy and feeling abandoned by her, just as he felt abandoned and stuck in his new home. She linked this back to his hidden feeling that others will find his presence unbearable and reject him, just as he found the other residents of the respite home unbearable. While Jack was still angry and initially refuted this interpretation, he was eventually able to endure the links made. Jack had reached Malan-stage 7 of therapy.

When Jack arrived for therapy the following week he appeared much calmer. In this and the following sessions, Jack was able to make secure links within the triangle of person, signifying that he had reached Malan-stage 8. He was able to link his fears of rejection to his inability to further his relationship with his ex-girlfriend. He acknowledged that his fears of intimacy stemmed from his father's rejection during his early years. Jack contemplated how this had led to his hidden feeling that he was unbearable and an unworthy person.

In Malan-stage 9, Jack was able to distance himself from his conflict suggesting that he was moving through a stage of resolution enhanced through a strengthened awareness of his past and present conflicts with other people in his life. One day he won football tickets and asked another man with ID from the respite home to go with him. It transpired that Jack and his housemate had been spending time together and struck up a friendship. Jack was also reported to be less withdrawn and able to accept support from the respite home staff around his personal affairs and care, which he had previously adamantly rejected.

In session 18, Jack was able to accept the termination of the therapy and said that he understood that the intervention had to come to an end so that the therapist could also provide interventions to other clients.

Evaluation of the case study

The above case study shows how PDT and a containing therapeutic experience can support the resolution of the ToC and ToP, and encourage the regression of the client to earlier developmental stages in order to experience the therapist's reaction as emotionally corrective (Alexander & French, 1946). By appreciating the therapist as reliable and engaged, hidden feelings of the 'unbearable' nature of Jack's presence, as well as anxieties over being rejected again, could be refuted, thus 'experiencing the old, unsettled conflict but with a new ending' (Alexander & French, 1946). In Kleinian terms, Jack has now reached the depressive position (Klein, 1952b), while Mahler *et al* (1975) would highlight his arrival at a stage of individuation.

Conclusion

This chapter has provided a brief outline of the complexities of PDT with people with ID, focusing on presentations of anxiety and depression, and different schools of thought have been explored to contextualise the treatment. Research in the area is scarce and lack of randomised control trials and controlled/comparative studies may be due to the lack of 'manualisation' of PDT. The above case study has shown that PDT can lead to an acceptance of the self and overcome the trauma of ID. Hollins and Evered (1990) suggested that discrepancy of ratings between real self and ideal self in people with ID widened during the first year of PDT as people were confronted with the reality of the ID and their defences increased. As treatment progressed, however, this discrepancy lessened and the gap closed in most cases.

PDT can make a valuable contribution towards the treatment of psychological disorders in people with ID and criticisms of the long term nature of PDT have been refuted by Beail *et al* (2007), who suggest that most change in PDT occurs within the first eight sessions. Further research to promote the evidence base of PDT is needed to promote its survival during times of change to the structure of the NHS and service provision.

Summary

- The use of PDT and deficits in self–other relating can explain the development of psychological difficulties such as anxiety and depressive disorders in people with ID.

- Attachment theory and previous primary care giver relationships, as well as current (carer) relationships, are taken into account when formulating cases from a psychodynamic perspective. This relational approach to formulation and treatment is intrinsic to PDT practice and distinguishes it from other ways of psychological working.

- PDT can enable patients to encounter corrective emotional experiences, allow them to become unstuck and progress in their emotional maturation.

References

Adler A (1927) *Understanding Human Nature*. Cited in J Clifford (1996) p114 op cit.

Alexander F & French T (1946) *Psychoanalytic Therapy*. New York: Ronald Press.

Applegate J & Barol B (1989) Repairing the nest: a psychodynamic developmental approach to clients with severe behaviour disorders. *Clinical Social Work Journal* **17** (3) 89–98.

Bachrach H & Leaf L (1978) Analyzability: a systemic review of the clinical and quantitative literature. *Journal of the American Psychoanalytic Association* **26** 881–920.

Beail N (1998) Psychoanalytic psychotherapy with men with intellectual disabilities: a preliminary outcome study. *Bristol Journal of Medical Psychology* **71** 1–11.

Beail N (2001) Recidivism following psychodynamic psychotherapy amongst offenders with intellectual disabilities. *The British Journal of Forensic Practice* **3** (1) 33–37.

Beail N (2003) What works for people with mental retardation? Critical commentary on cognitive-behavioural and psychodynamic psychotherapy research. *Mental Retardation* **41** (6) 468–472.

Beail N, Kellett S, Newman D & Warden S (2007) The dose effect relationship in psychodynamic psychotherapy with people with intellectual disabilities. *Journal of Applied Research in Intellectual Disabilities* **20** (5) 448–454.

Beail N & Warden S (1996) Sexual abuse of adults with learning disabilities. *Journal of Intellectual Disability Research* **39** (5) 382–387.

Bowlby J (1979) *The Making and Breaking of Affectional Bonds*. London: Tavistock Publications.

Carlson D (1979) Affective psychosis in mental retardates. *Psychiatric Clinics of North America* **2** 499–509.

Carlson E, Sampson M & Sroufe L (2003) Attachment theory and pediatric practice. *Journal of Developmental and Behavioural Pediatrics* **24** (5) 364–379.

Clegg J & Sheard C (2002) Challenging behaviour and insecure attachment. *Journal of Intellectual Disability Research* **46** (6) 503–506.

Clifford J (1996) Adlerian therapy. In: W Dryden (Ed) *Handbook of Individual Therapy*. London: Sage.

Cooper C (1996) Psychodynamic Therapy: The Kleinian approach. In: W Dryden (Ed) *Handbook of Individual Therapy*. London: Sage.

Dodd P & McGinnity M (2003) Psychotherapy and Learning Disability. *Irish Journal of Psychiatric Medicine* **20** (2) 38–40.

Donovan C & Spence S (2000) Prevention of childhood anxiety disorders. *Clinical Psychology Review* **20** (4) 509–531.

Dryden W (1996) *Handbook of Individual Therapy*. London: Sage.

Einfeld S & Aman M (1995) Issues in the taxonomy of psychopathology of mental retardation. *Journal of Autism and Developmental Disorders* **25** (2) 143–167.

Frankish P (1989) Meeting the emotional needs of handicapped people: a psycho-dynamic approach. *Journal of Mental Deficiency Research* **33** (5) 407–414.

Freud S (1893) In: J Strachey (Ed) *Standard Edition of the Complete Psychological Works of Sigmund Freud, Vol 2*. London: Hogarth Press.

Freud S (1905) Three essays on the theory of sexuality. In: J Strachey (Ed) *The Standard Edition of the Complete Psychological Works of Sigmund Freud, Vol 7: 'A Case of Hysteria', 'Three Essays on Sexuality' and other works*. New York: W W Norton and Company.

Freud S (1923) Neurosis and psychosis. In: J Strachey (Ed) *The Standard Edition of the Complete Psychological Works of Sigmund Freud, Vol 19: 'The Ego and the Id' and other works*. New York: W W Norton and Company.

Gerhardt S (2004) *Why Love Matters: How affection shapes a baby's brain*. London: Routledge.

Hollins S & Evered C (1990) Group process and content: the challenge of mental handicap. *Group Analysis* **23** (1) 56–67.

Hollins S & Sinason V (2000) Psychotherapy, learning disabilities and trauma: new perspectives. *British Journal of Psychiatry* **176** 32–36.

Jacobs M (2004) *Psychodynamic Counselling in Action* (3rd edition). London: Sage.

Klein M (1952a) Notes on some schizoid mechanisms. In: J Riviere (Ed) *Developments in Psycho-Analysis*. London: Hogarth Press.

Klein M (1952b) On the theory of anxiety and guilt. In: J Riviere (Ed) *Developments in Psycho-analysis*. London: Hogarth Press.

Klein M (1960) *Our Adult World and its Roots in Infancy*. London: Tavistock.

Klein M (1975) *Love, Guilt and Reparation*. London: Hogarth Press.

Kovacs M (1985) The children's depression inventory. *Psychopharmacology Bulletin* **21** (4) 995–998.

Leichsenring F, Hiller W, Weissberg M & Leibing E (2006) Cognitive-behavioral therapy and psychodynamic psychotherapy: techniques, efficacy, and indications. *American Journal of Psychotherapy* **60** (3) 233–259.

Lund J (1985) The prevalence of psychiatric morbidity in mentally retarded adults. *Acta Psychiatrica Scandinavica* **72** (6) 563–570.

Malan D (1979) *Individual Psychotherapy and the Science of Psychodynamics*. London: Butterworth.

Mahler M, Pines F & Bergman A (1975) *The Psychological Birth of the Human Infant*. New York: Basic Books, Inc.

Mannoni M (1972) *The Backward Child and His Mother: A psychoanalytic study*. New York: Pantheon Books.

McDonald M (1970) Transitional tunes and musical development. *Psychoanalytic Study of the Child* **25** 503–520.

Menninger K (1958) *Theory of Psychoanalytic Technique*. New York: Basic Books.

Menolascino F (1965) Emotional disturbance and mental retardation. *American Journal of Mental Deficiency* **70** (2) 248–56.

Meins W (1993) Assessment of depression in mentally retarded adults: reliability and validity of the Children's Depression Inventory (CDI). *Research in Developmental Disabilities* **14** (4) 299–312.

Miller A (1983) *For Your Own Good*. London: Virago Press.

Myers B (1986) Psychopathology in hospitalised developmentally disabled individuals. *Comprehensive Psychiatry* **27** (2) 115–126.

Neal J & Edelmann R (2003) The etiology of social phobia: toward a developmental profile. *Clinical Psychology Review* **23** (6) 761–786.

Parloff M, Kelman H & Frank J (1954) Comfort, effectiveness and self-awareness as criteria of improvement in psychotherapy. *American Journal of Psychiatry* **111** (5) 343–352.

Prout H & Nowak-Drabik K (2003) Psychotherapy with persons who have mental retardation: an evaluation of effectiveness. *American Journal of Mental Retardation* **108** (2) 82–93.

Reed J (1997) Understanding and assessing depression in people with learning disabilities: a cognitive-behavioural approach. In: B Kroese, D Dagnan and K Loumidis (Eds) *Cognitive Behaviour Therapy for People with Learning Disabilities*. London: Routledge.

Reiss S, Levitan G & McNally R (1982) Emotionally disturbed mentally retarded people: an underserved population. *American Psychologist* **37** (4) 361–367.

Roth A & Fonagy P (2006) *What Works for Whom: A critical review of psychotherapy research* (2nd edition). London: Guilford Press.

Scotti J, Evans I, Meyer I & Walker P (1991) A meta-analysis of intervention research with problem behavior: treatment validity and standard of practice. *American Journal of Mental Retardation* **96** (3) 233–256.

Sinason V (1992) *Mental Handicap and the Human Condition: New approaches from the Tavistock*. London: Free Association Books.

Smith D (1996) Psychodynamic Therapy: The Freudian approach. In: W Dryden (Ed) *Handbook of Individual Therapy*. London: Sage.

Sovner R & Hurley R (1981) The management of chronic behaviour disorders in mentally retarded adults with lithium carbonate. *The Journal of Nervous and Mental Disease* **69** (3)

191–5.

Stoddart K (1996) *Knowledge of Bereavement and Death Questionnaire*. Unpublished questionnaire. Cited in Stoddart *et al* (2002) p31 op cit.

Stoddart K, Burke L & Temple V (2002) Outcome evaluation of bereavement groups for adults with intellectual disabilities. *Journal of Applied Research in Intellectual Disabilities* **15** (1) 28–35.

Sturmey P (2004) Cognitive therapy with people with intellectual disabilities: a selective review and critique. *Clinical Psychology and Psychotherapy* **11** (4) 222–232.

Turner R (2000) fMRI: methodology–sensimotor function mapping. *Advanced Neurology* **83** 213–220.

Wallerstein R (1987) The assessment of analyzability and of analytic outcomes. *Yearbook of Psychoanalysis and Psychotherapy* **2** 416–427.

Warren S, Huston L, Egeland B & Sroufe L (1997) Child and adolescent anxiety disorders and attachment. *American Academy of Child and Adolescent Psychiatry* **36** (5) 637–644.

Willner P (2005) The effectiveness of psychotherapeutic interventions for people with learning disabilities: a critical overview. *Journal of Intellectual Disability Research* **49** (1) 73–85.

Winnicott D (1958) *Collected Papers: Through paediatrics to psychoanalysis.* London: Hogarth Press.

Winnicott D (1965) Failure of expectable environment on child's mental functioning. *International Journal of Psychoanalysis* **46** 81–87.

Winnicott D (1970) On the basis of self in the body. In: C Winnicott, R Shepherd and M Davis (Eds) (1989) *Psychoanalytic Explorations*. London: Karnac.

Yalom I (1985) *The Theory and Practice of Group Psychotherapy*. New York: Basic Books.

Zigler E, Bennett-Gates D, Hodapp R & Henrich C (2002) Assessing personality traits of individuals with mental retardation. *American Journal on Mental Retardation* **107** (3) 181–193.

Chapter 10

Supporting families

Ereny Gobrial and Raghu Raghavan

Overview

This chapter focuses on supporting the families of children and young people with ID, autism and anxiety. A parent support model for managing the anxiety of this group will be explored, and its implementation on a small group of parents will be discussed.

Learning objectives

- To understand the co-morbidity of ID, autism and anxiety.
- To develop a programme of anxiety management strategies.
- To examine the effectiveness of a parental programme.

Introduction

There is growing evidence that children with autism and ID have higher rates of co-morbid psychiatric disorders than typically developing children, including anxiety disorders and depression (Brown, 2000; Brereton *et al*, 2006). Studies show that, for both adults and adolescents, those with both ID and autism have higher levels of anxiety than groups with ID but not autism (Hill & Furniss, 2006; Bradley *et al*, 2004). In young people with autism, anxiety is significantly higher than in young people with ID without autism (Brereton *et al*, 2006). In fact, epidemiological studies estimate that the prevalence of anxiety in children and young people with autism ranges from 13.6% to 84% (Muris & Steerneman, 1998; Gillott *et al*, 2001; Sukhodolsky *et al*, 2008; Simmonoff *et al*, 2008).

It is important to note that anxiety disorder is more likely to increase during the transition from childhood to teenager, and this is a stage when they are most vulnerable to develop mental health problems in general (FPLD, 2005). Growing up is a very difficult and stressful period for many young people and adolescents, and it may be even more stressful for young people with ID who are not fully aware of the process of change and who are faced with making choices about the future and their aspirations (Raghavan & Pawson, 2008). They are, for example, more likely to be worried about bodily appearance or about leaving home than their peers (Graham, 1991), and there are other changes that can affect them, especially the loss of friends or social networks, which can put them at greater risk of developing mental health problems (Raghavan & Pawson, 2008). Furthermore, it is also possible that as children grow older they are better able to express their emotions and their parents become better observers of anxiety disorder, or these symptoms become more prominent in the home (Weisbrot *et al*, 2005) leading to a greater incidence of reported cases than in younger children.

It is recognised that emotional problems such as anxiety disorder occur frequently in young people with autism as a consequence of the features that define the condition (Leyfer *et al*, 2006), such as low intellectual abilities, poor communication skills, a lack of social and cognitive resources and poor coping skills (particularly for higher functioning individuals who are more aware of the difficulties and challenges they face). For example:

- low intellectual abilities and poor cognitive skills are more likely to lead to low self-esteem (Henry & Crabbe, 2002)
- a lack of communication skills may result in greater difficulties in discussing or dismissing fears, resulting in over-generalisation (Smiley, 2005)
- poor coping skills may result in greater anxiety as children face unfamiliar problem-solving tasks (Henry & Crabbe, 2002).

Furthermore, other deficits associated with autism, such as difficulty in understanding emotions and interpersonal relations, along with misinterpretation of social cues, may also lead to anxiety disorder.

It is also important to note that sensory integration affects a significant number of individuals with autism (Rogers *et al*, 2003) and research shows that sensory processing is related to autism symptoms and anxiety disorder. People with autism often experience forms of sensory sensitivity, either hyper-sensitive or hypo-sensitive (Aron & Aron, 1997), which can impact greatly on their behaviour and contribute to anxiety disorder (Sofronoff *et al*, 2005).

In brief, all of the above factors suggest that the co-morbidity of ID and autism results in an increased vulnerability to anxiety disorder.

The impact on families

Experiencing significant levels of anxiety can be disabling for children with autism and ID, resulting in negative consequences for both the children themselves and their families. Anxiety may cause considerable distress, interfere with a child's daily activities (Muris & Steerneman, 1998; Bellini, 2004) and further impede their interactions with others (Rapee *et al*, 2008), and evidence shows that a child's emotional and behavioural difficulties has a significant impact on family well-being (Herring *et al*, 2006; Tehee *et al*, 2009). In fact, caring for a child with autism and ID can make parents themselves more vulnerable to developing mental health disorders, such as stress or depression, than other parents (Hastings *et al*, 2006; Heiman, 2002; Grant *et al*, 1998).

Parents are generally considered to be a child's most important resource, and they have a vital role to play in providing the support that a child needs. However, we often tend to ignore or marginalise the role of family carers in interventions at home, but in fact parental involvement in interventions with children with autism and/or ID is an important ingredient in ensuring positive outcomes (Diggle *et al*, 2008; Ozonoff & Cathcart, 1998). It is suggested that the majority of family carers can give better care than anyone else, and Grant *et al* (1998) point out that '*services have many things to learn from family caregivers*' (p46).

Despite this, there is little published research attempting to develop parental interventions that address anxiety in children and young people who are diagnosed with both autism and ID. Almost all published studies in this area address psychosocial interventions (eg. Chalfant *et al*, 2007; Reaven & Hepburn, 2003; Sofronoff *et al*, 2005). Given the importance of involving parents, and the fact that parental support has received little attention in the management of anxiety in children and young people with autism and ID, this chapter will examine a family carer intervention model known as the Calm Child Programme (CCP), for children and young people with ID, autism and anxiety disorders.

CCP

There is an abundance of literature about family intervention and early intervention programmes for autism in children, such as the Son-Rise programme and Applied Behaviour Analysis (ABA). These programmes encourage many positive improvements for families, such as enhancing parents' confidence, relieving parental stress, cost effectiveness, enhancing the capacity of the family, and increasing quality of life (Grant *et al*, 1998). The CCP was specifically designed for parents who have a child or adolescent with ID and autism and was developed in consultation with parents, teachers and a group of professionals working in the field of child and adolescent mental health. A study was conducted with these groups to explore the range of anxiety management strategies used by parents and teachers. These strategies were then further discussed with professionals to develop a model of the types of interventions that are useful and which can easily be implemented by parents, to provide them with effective and practical management strategies to help children and young people manage and cope with anxiety.

Program content and components

The programme consists of three types of management strategy that, at different levels, were intended to complement each other:

- Proactive strategies: these aim at crisis prevention, and are recommended for use on a daily basis to prevent triggering anxiety by using visual schedules, talking and explaining, relaxation techniques and physical activities.
- Communication strategies: these aim to communicate with the child or young person when they begin to feel anxious using an 'anxiety scale thermometer' that helps to identify the level of a child's anxiety so that parents can implement appropriate strategies from the 'traffic light system' used by the CCP.
- Reactive strategies: these are designed to manage the child's anxiety, using distraction, 'quiet time', fun activities and comfort strategies. These are recommended when a child shows behaviours related to severe anxiety.

The CCP consists of two parts; one providing basic information about autism and anxiety, and the other covering simple anxiety management strategies. What follows is an extract from the CCP.

Part 1:
What do you know about autism, intellectual disabilities, and anxiety?

Children with autism show three types of symptoms:

- impaired social interaction
- problems with verbal and nonverbal communication and imagination
- unusual or severely limited activities and interests.

Intellectual disability includes the presence of a significantly reduced ability to understand new or complex information or to learn new skills (impaired intelligence), with a reduced ability to cope independently (impaired social functioning) that started before adulthood, with a lasting effect on development?

Anxiety: what is it?

All children experience some anxiety. This is normal and expected, but when it interrupts a child's normal activities such as attending school and making friends or sleeping, and has a bad impact on their overall adaptation behaviour, such anxiety becomes a problem.

How do children with autism spectrum disorders show anxiety?

Children and young people with autism experience a wide variety of fears and anxiety.

Children are all different:

- they might feel very hot or sweaty
- they may cry a lot
- they may shake hands and legs
- they might feel breathless
- they might find it is difficult to sit still
- they might feel panicky
- their stomach might feel funny.

Children with autism also feel worried or nervous in different ways.

Here are some words or phrases that children with autism and learning disabilities might use to explain their fears and worries:

- stressed
- things wrong with me
- fed up

- frightened
- in a temper
- in a huff.

What can cause anxiety?

There are lots of reasons why children and young people may be at risk of getting nervous:

- when you change their daily routine
- when they meet new people
- when someone comes to your house
- when they are in busy or crowded places
- when facing new or unexpected situations
- when they are worried about family, the future or their mental health
- difficulties in understanding the world and in communicating with others.

Part 2:

Anxiety management strategies

What are anxiety management strategies?

Anxiety management strategies involve techniques that parents and teachers can use to help children with autism and learning disabilities to cope better with their worries and fears. This information sheet shows you some management strategies that parents and teachers think are useful for managing anxiety in children and young people with autism. Professionals such as psychiatrists, psychologists, nurses and social workers have also seen these strategies and think they could be useful.

We operate a 'traffic light' system to determine a child's level of anxiety and to show how you can help them to cope with each level. GREEN refers to strategies you might use most of the time when your child is OK. AMBER represents strategies that you might use once you notice that your child is becoming anxious. Finally, RED represents strategies you should use when he is anxious (Figure 10.1).

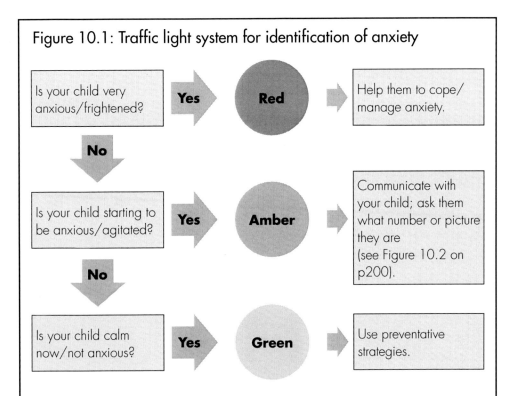

Figure 10.1: Traffic light system for identification of anxiety

Is your child very anxious/frightened? — **Yes** → **Red** → Help them to cope/manage anxiety.

No

Is your child starting to be anxious/agitated? — **Yes** → **Amber** → Communicate with your child; ask them what number or picture they are (see Figure 10.2 on p200).

No

Is your child calm now/not anxious? — **Yes** → **Green** → Use preventative strategies.

Daily life strategies

The green light strategy is a proactive approach that aims at crisis prevention. The focus is on supporting your child to remain calm, and helping you to remain one step ahead. You might need to use these ideas most of the time, day by day, in order to reduce your child's anxiety. Here are some recommended ideas:

Visual schedule

The visual schedule or timetable uses pictures as a means of supporting your child to cope with change. Children with autism are more sensitive to any change in their daily routine, and so this visual timetable helps to reduce anxiety because it helps them to understand what they are going to do during their day. A visual timetable makes time concrete, allows a child to see time passing, and to understand plans for the future.

For most children, the timetable should be arranged from left to right. For some young children, a top to bottom format may be more understandable.

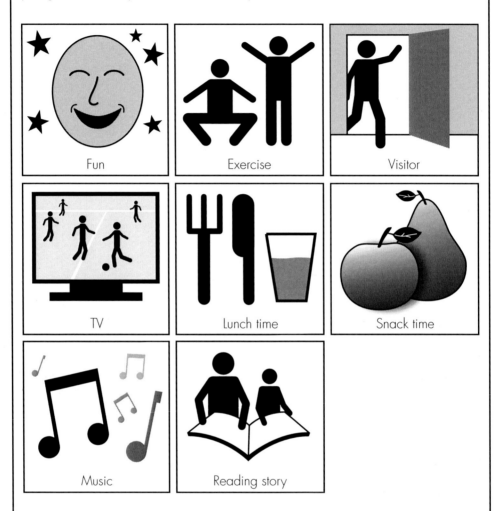

Fun	Exercise	Visitor
TV	Lunch time	Snack time
Music	Reading story	

Talking and explaining

Always talk to your child, in very simple language, about what they are going to do. Keep the information very simple. Talk about the situation and let your child know what is happening. For example, suggestions like, 'we are now eating a snack, and then in five minutes we will play' or 'in half an hour we will put on our coats and shoes on and we will get in the car'. The basic rule is to be clear, concise, and consistent.

Anxiety and Depression in People with Intellectual Disabilities   © Pavilion Publishing and Media Ltd 2012

Explain in advance any events that are out of your child's usual routine. You could, for example, use leaflets or brochures to explain holidays or school trips.

Regular physical activities

Physical activity is very good for your child, particularly if they are very agitated. Activities that other parents have found helpful are:

- getting outside and doing some exercise, such as running in the garden or swinging
- going for a walk – a short walk in the fresh air can help improve a child's mood, or perhaps a long walk with the dog
- jumping on a trampoline
- special regular activities such as swimming, karate, horse riding, football or dancing.

Relaxation

Help your child to relax. First, it is important to create a relaxing environment so choose a comfortable, quiet and peaceful room. It may be possible to teach your child how to relax as a coping skill when they become agitated or angry. There are many ways to help them to relax including:

- Breathing techniques: teach them to take the time to breathe slowly and deeply, and count from one to 10, as this can help promote a feeling of calmness. Also practice some breathing exercises, for example, ask your child to pretend that they are blowing up a balloon and then letting the balloon out.
- Listening to relaxing music: music can stimulate and develop more meaningful and playful communication in people with autism. It can also play an important role for children with autism in developing positive interactions. For example, you can use calming music every night before bedtime.
- Reading books: for example, a book explaining to the child how they can express their feelings.
- Having a warm bath in low lighting.

Communicate with your child's anxiety

It is essential to talk to your child and to gain their views on certain situations. Children may be able describe their fears or anxieties, as well as the situations that give rise to them. This communication is likely to be helpful. If you notice your child becoming worried or agitated, then there is an opportunity to start to communicate with them. You might therefore tell them that you have noticed that they look anxious, for example, by asking them how they feel.

Thermometer approach

You may present the 'thermometer of anxiety' rating scale to your child and ask them to let you know which number they are at (see Figure 10.2).

For example, you might ask, 'how worried are you? Can you show me? Are you a two or a three?'

Figure 10.2: Anxiety thermometer

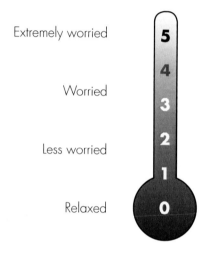

Anxiety pictures/numbers

You can use pictures to help your child tell you about their feelings. You might ask your child to draw pictures that make sense to them.

Example 1

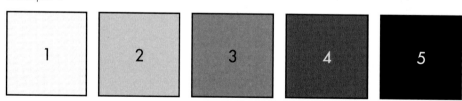

Example 2

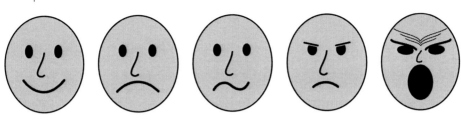

Reactive strategies

When your child is agitated or feeling anxious, there are a number of ways to help them to cope with anxiety.

- Have a little fun. Having fun or playing is a great way to improve mood and release tension, although it is often easier for children than for adolescents. For example, you might play their favourite games or try some painting.

- Special interest (distractive). One way of helping your child to cope with their anxiety is to make use of their particular interests. When you find that your child is agitated, ignore the situation and try to distract them before their anxiety level escalates. The trick here is to let them do something they enjoy, such as watching DVDs, playing favourite games, jumping, drawing, feeding the birds or getting out their favourite toys.

- Quiet time out. Time out gives your child the chance to manage themselves and to calm down. The amount of time given should be kept brief, between one to three minutes for each episode, although this can be repeated. A quiet stimulation-free spot is a good choice. Some children ask for time out for themselves.

- Comfort strategy (reassurance and cuddling). Parents can offer physical expressions of love for their child to help to calm them down. Simply placing your hands on their back or holding hands can be very relaxing. You will know what areas are most sensitive for your child and so avoid them. You may need to find out what sort of touch or holding gives most comfort.

Implementation of the CCP

In order to implement the CCP, a pilot study was conducted over three months with seven families with children with autism and ID to evaluate its use. First, a meeting was organised with parents in order to explain about the CCP information pack. This information pack included:

- the CCP itself
- the Glasgow Anxiety Scale (GAS-ID) (Mindham & Espie, 2003)
- a parents' dairy
- consent forms
- an example of a visual schedule.

All participating parents gave their written consent for their participation before the start of the programme, and they completed the GAS-ID. They were then asked to monitor their children on a daily basis and record in a diary the levels of anxiety observed, any related behaviours and which of the above strategies they used to address the problems and their various outcomes. Parents were contacted every two weeks to get an update on how they were experiencing the CCP. At the end of the implementation period of three months, parents completed another GAS-ID about their child and an evaluation form about the programme. A focus group was then organised to discuss the usefulness of using the various management strategies.

85% of participating children and young people showed statistically significant improvements in anxiety levels between pre- and post-test. Furthermore, parents who implemented the programme were more likely to manage their child's anxiety more positively.

The focus group emphasised the effectiveness of the CCP in managing children's anxiety, and it was discovered that the most effective strategies were talking and explaining, physical activities and distraction. The majority of parents used a combination of these different strategies to manage the child's anxiety, however it is interesting that the parents also reported that the children began to self-manage using the same strategies when they were feeling stressed or worried.

A strong theme that emerged from the CCP was that it improved parents' confidence and increased their knowledge and skills in recognising and managing anxiety. The CCP supports parents to manage the anxiety of children and young people with autism and ID, enhancing family protective factors and reducing risk factors associated with severe emotional difficulties. The parental programme can also help reduce parents' anxiety, and the high levels of stress they may experience, especially within the parenting role (Tehee *et al*, 2009; White & Hastings, 2004). Providing parents with a practical and appropriate programme of parental strategies helps to strengthen the family's capacity to meet the needs of the child (Wang *et al*, 2006). Prevention programmes starting in early childhood can improve outcomes for children and families and providing a programme to support parents to manage their child's anxiety is likely to reduce the demand for services, both for the child and the parent, resulting in a reduction in service costs and workloads for professionals (Mudford *et al*, 2001; Smith *et al*, 2000).

Conclusion

A simple and easy to use intervention strategy, the CCP was developed for addressing anxiety in children and young people with autism and ID. The implementation of the CCP showed that management strategies and interventions targeting children and young people with autism and ID were effective, and that involving the parents in interventions is a successful model for caring for this group. Supporting families in the implementation of intervention strategies will put them in control and develop their confidence when caring for children with ID, autism and anxiety.

Summary

- Children with intellectual disabilities and autism experience higher levels of anxiety. This has a significant impact on the well-being of the family.

- An intervention strategy known as the Calm Child Programme has been developed for parents to manage the anxiety of their children with ID and autism. A pilot study of this intervention strategy indicates a significant improvement in anxiety levels for children with ID and autism.

References

Aron E & Aron A (1997) Sensory-processing sensitivity and its relation to introversion and emotionality. *Journal of Personality and Social Psychology* **73** (2) 345–368.

Bellini S (2004) Social skill deficits and anxiety in high functioning adolescents with autism spectrum disorders. *Focus on Autism and Other Developmental Disabilities* **19** (2) 78–86.

Bradley E, Summers J, Wood H & Bryson S (2004) Comparing rates of psychiatric and behaviour disorders in adolescents and young adults with severe intellectual disability with and without autism. *Journal of Autism & Developmental Disorders* **34** (2) 151–161.

Brereton A, Tonge B & Einfeld S (2006) Psychopathology in children and adolescents with autism compared to young people with intellectual disability. *Journal of Autism and Developmental Disorders* **36** (7) 863–870.

Brown G (2000) Medical sociology and issues of aetiology. In: M Gleder, J Lopez-Ibor and N Andeason (Eds) *Textbook of Psychiatry*. Oxford: Oxford University press.

Chalfant A, Rappee R & Carroll L (2007) Treating anxiety disorders in children with high functioning autism spectrum disorders: a controlled trial. *Journal of Autism and Developmental Disorders* **37** (10) 1842–1857.

Diggle T, McConachie H & Randle V (2008) Parents-mediated early intervention for young children with autism spectrum disorder (review). *Cochran Database of Systematic Reviews* (1) CD003496.

Foundation for People with Learning Disabilities (FPLD) (2005) *Making Us Count: Identifying and improving mental health support for young people with learning disabilities*. London: The mental Health Foundation.

Gillott A, Furniss F & Walter A (2001) Anxiety in high-functioning children with autism. *Autism* **5** (3) 277–286.

Graham P (1991) *Child Psychiatry: A developmental approach* (2nd edition). Oxford: Oxford medical publication.

Grant G, Ramcharan P, McGrath M, Nolan M & Keady J (1998) Rewards and gratifications among family caregivers: towards a refined model of caring and coping. *Journal of Intellectual Disability Research* **42** (1) 58–71.

Hastings R, Daley D, Burns C & Beck A (2006) Maternal distress and expressed emotion: cross-sectional and longitudinal relationships with behaviour problems of children with intellectual disabilities. *American Journal of Mental Retardation* **111** (1) 48–61.

Heiman T (2002) Parents of children with disabilities: resilience, coping and future expectations. *Journal of Developmental and Physical Disabilities* **14** (2) 156–171.

Henry F & Crabbe M (2002) Treatment of anxiety disorders in persons with mental retardation. In: A Dosen and K Day (Eds) *Treating Mental Illness and Behaviour Disorders in Children and Adults With Mental Retardation* (pp227). Arlington, VA: American Psychiatric Press.

Herring S, Gray K, Tonge T, Sweeney D & Einfeld S (2006) Behaviour and emotional problems in toddlers with pervasive developmental disorders and developmental delay: associations with parental mental health and family functioning. *Journal of Intellectual Disability Research* **50** (12) 874–882.

Hill J & Furniss F (2006) Patterns of emotional and behavioural disturbance associated with autistic traits in young people with severe intellectual disabilities and challenging behaviours. *Research in Developmental Disabilities* **27** (5) 517–528.

Leyfer O, Folstein S, Bacalman S, Davis N, Dinh E, Morgan J, Tager-Flusberg H & Lainhart J (2006) Comorbid psychiatric disorders in children with autism: interview development and rates of disorders. *Journal of Autism and Developmental Disorders* **36** (7) 849–861.

Mindham J & Espie C (2003) Glasgow Anxiety Scale for people with an intellectual disability (GAS-ID): development and psychometric properties of a new measure for use with people with mild intellectual disability. *Journal of Intellectual Disability Research* **47** (1) 22–30.

Mudford O, Martin N, Eikeseth S & Bibby P (2001) Parent-managed behavioral treatment for preschool children with autism: some characteristics of UK programs. *Research in Developmental Disabilities* **22** (3) 173–182.

Muris P & Steerneman P (1998) Comorbid anxiety symptoms in children with pervasive developmental disorders. *Journal of Anxiety disorders* **12** (4) 387–393.

Ozonoff S & Cathcart K (1998) Effectiveness of a home program intervention for young children with autism. *Journal of Autism and Developmental Disorders* **28** (1) 25–32.

Raghavan R & Pawson N (2008) Transition and social networks of young people with learning disabilities. *Advances in Mental Health and Learning Disabilities* **2** (3) 25–28.

Rapee R, Psych A, Spence S, Cobham V & Lyneham H (2008) *Helping Your Anxious Child* (2nd edition). Oakland, CA: New Harbinger.

Reaven J & Hepburn S (2003) Cognitive-behavioural treatment of obsessive-compulsive disorder in a child with Asperger's syndrome: a case report. *Autism* **7** (2) 145–164.

Rogers S, Hepburn S & Wehner E (2003) Parent reports of sensory symptoms in toddlers with autism and those with other developmental disorders. *Journal of Autism and Developmental Disorders* **33** (6) 631.

Simmonoff E, Pickles A, Charman T, Chandler S, Loucas T & Baird G (2008) Psychiatric disorders in children with autism spectrum disorders: Prevalence, comorbidity, and associated factors in a population-derived sample. *Journal of the American Academy of Child and Adolescent Psychiatry* **47** (8) 921–929.

Smiley E (2005) Epidemiology of mental health problems in adults with learning disability: an update. *Advances in Psychiatric Treatment* **11** 214–222.

Smith T, Buch G & Gamby T (2000) Parent-directed, intensive early intervention for children with pervasive developmental disabilities. *Research in Developmental Disabilities* **21** (4) 297–309.

Sofronoff K, Attwood T & Hinton S (2005) A randomised controlled trial of a CBT intervention for anxiety in children with Asperger's syndrome. *Journal of Child Psychology and Psychiatry* **46** (11) 1152–1160.

Sukhodolsky D, Scahill L, Gadow K, Arnold L, Aman M, McDougle C, McCracken J, Tierney E, Williams W, Lecavalier L & Vitiello B (2008) Parent-Rated anxiety symptoms in children with pervasive developmental disorders: frequency and association with core autism symptoms and cognitive functioning. *Journal of Abnormal Child Psychology* **36** (1) 117–128.

Tehee E, Honan R & Hevey D (2009) Factors contributing to stress in parents of individuals with autistic spectrum disorders. *Journal of Applied Research in Developmental Disabilities* **22** (1) 34–42.

Wang M, Summer J, Little T, Turnbull A, Poston D & Mannan H (2006) Perspectives of fathers and mothers of children in early intervention programmes in assessing family quality of life. *Journal of Intellectual Disability Research* **50** (12) 977–988.

Weisbrot D, Gadow K, DeVincent C & Pomeroy J (2005) The presentation of anxiety in children with pervasive developmental disorders. *Journal of Child Adolescent Psychopharmacology* **15** (3) 477–496.

White N & Hastings N (2004) Social and professional support for parents of adolescents with severe intellectual disabilities. *Journal of Applied Research in Intellectual Disabilities* **17** (3) 181–190.

Chapter 11

Case management and the care programme approach

Eddie Chaplin and Steve Hardy

Overview

This chapter provides a brief history of the theories and development of case management and the care programme approach (CPA) within mental health services. It examines how these approaches have been used to benefit the care of people with ID by the use of case examples.

Learning objectives

- To have an overview of community mental health care models.
- To understand the CPA from its development to how it is currently implemented.
- To be able to be able to understand community mental health care and the CPA as it relates to people with ID, in particular those with anxiety and depression.

Introduction

The case management model has evolved over time, adapting to the changing times and the needs of local populations. In many areas changes to the model have led to different levels of service being provided. Community mental health services have been described and configured in a number of ways (eg. standard community treatment, assertive outreach, case management, intensive case management), however a lack of standard definitions mean that often these terms are interchangeable.

Case management has largely moved away from philosophy-driven models and is more likely to be defined by the presence of common characteristics. Two examples that try to describe case management using common characteristics are:

- *'any systematic or structured management of patient care that included co-ordination and communication among treating health care providers, patient education, monitoring of symptoms and adherence to treatment plans, self-management support or psychological treatments'* (Williams *et al*, 2007).
- Intagliata (1982) offers five underlying principles to define case management (based on Agranoff, 1977), revised below:
  - detailed assessment of individual's needs
  - development of care packages tailored to the individual
  - ensuring access to these services
  - monitoring the quality of services
  - offering long-term flexible support, which is adjusted to the individual's needs.

In 1954, Warlingham Park Hospital established the first community roles for mental health nurses. Initially, this was by providing outpatient services, and the role later developed to include visiting and supporting people who had just left hospital, not only with their mental health symptoms but also with employment, accommodation and other areas that impact on mental well-being (Moore, 1960, 1964).

The first use of case management in clinical practice was in the US, which was designed to help people live in the community and reduce the rates of hospital admission. In the late 1960s, the Madison model of community care was developed by Stein and Test (1980), although there were few community facilities apart from some day hospitals and halfway houses for people with serious mental illnesses (Thompson *et al*, 1990).

In the 1970s, the Training in Community Living Programme was introduced, known later as the Program of Assertive Community Treatment (PACT). This is widely accepted to be the first model of assertive community treatment, and it set the standard for assertive outreach services as a viable alternative to treatment in a mental hospital. The PACT service still exists today and aims to provide 24-hour care directly to people as part of a community multidisciplinary team, working with people in their own homes. Central to its philosophy is the need to move away from traditional service user roles by addressing the people's needs in all areas of their lives, such as employment, accommodation, daily activities, shopping and self-care.

In the UK, the first trial of assertive outreach or intensive home-based treatment (which is considered case management) was conducted by Muijen *et al* (1992) in South London. This was called the Daily Living Programme (DLP) and was evaluated as part of a randomised controlled trial. The DLP was staffed mainly by psychiatrists, nurses and occupational therapists, and the study reported dramatic decreases in the number of hospital admissions. Since then there have been a number of similar studies, however findings have been difficult to generalise because of differences in methodology, for example service design, interfaces between services, commissioning patterns, changing needs of the population and definitions of case management. Another reason why case management is not a uniform concept is because it has been developed using different philosophies to meet a wide range of needs. Examples of the different models are listed in Table 11.1 on p210.

Evidence from studies

The variation in definitions of community interventions has led to studies being criticised, including the largest ever study in the UK (UK 700, Burns *et al*, 1999) because the services studied did not meet the minimum definition of intensive case management (see Smith & Newton, 2007).

Marshall *et al* (1998), as part of a Cochrane review focused on assertive community, reported that case management shortens the length of hospital admissions. A more recent review, however, (Smith & Newton, 2007) reported mixed results, suggesting that there is a gap between case management and standard community treatment, although there is evidence to suggest that this gap is closing and that both approaches are best studied together.

Table 11.1: Case management models	
Case management models	Purpose
Madison model	This was the founder of the assertive outreach approach and viewed patients as citizens who had a right to be integrated into society. This was achieved by providing material resources, retaining responsibility for care with the aim of giving the motivation to persevere.
Personal strengths model	The personal strengths model looks at an individual's strengths and aims to build upon these by offering a titrated service so those in need will get most input or those most at threat of hospitalisation. There is less of a risk of becoming dependent. Like the Madison model, it views patients as citizens and uses professionals as well as para-professionals.
Clinical case management model	The clinical case management model seeks to empower the patient by exploring relationships within a psychodynamic framework that explores relationships.
Rehabilitation orientated model	The rehab-orientated model suggests that there is a disease process that is at the route of any disintegrative process. It also implies goals and achievements through the use of the medical model and behavioural interventions.

Muijen *et al* (1992), meanwhile, reported that there was no difference in the outcomes achieved by generic community psychiatric nurses compared to case managers in relation to the number of admissions, the length of stay, psychopathology, patient satisfaction and social functioning.

In examining the effectiveness of case management and more generic community treatment for people with ID, there is little evidence to suggest one approach over another with no substantial evidence base to draw upon and even less if we were to look for evidence for the use of case management in this group for depression and anxiety specifically. The UK700 project (Hassiotis *et al*, 1999) examined the implementation of case management with patients with psychoses. Part of this project examined a subgroup of people with lower intellectual functioning (those with an IQ between 71–85) (Hassiotis *et al*, 1999), and the results, published two years later, showed reductions in days spent in hospital, the number of hospital admissions and increased user satisfaction for the group with borderline intellectual functioning compared to other groups (Hassiotis *et al*, 2001).

Some studies have focused on depression in the general population, and in primary care systematic reviews have shown promising results. In a review of 28 studies of case management for depression, 20 people were found to have improved outcomes over a 12-month period, giving good evidence that supports the use of short-term case management (Williams *et al*, 2007). In another review of 13 studies, case management was reported to have improved the management of major depression in primary healthcare settings (Genischen *et al*, 2005).

In terms of the delivery of services, a study of healthcare assistants in Germany using a clustered randomised control trial (Genischen *et al*, 2009) reported that a case management approach may produce better outcomes in terms of reducing symptoms and the way care is delivered.

The CPA

In England, the CPA has incorporated case management principles for those felt to be most at risk to themselves or others, regardless of their diagnosis. In reality, the CPA has formalised the use of case management (Simpson *et al*, 2003) and inter agency co-operation between services by providing a framework within which to work. The CPA was introduced following a number of high-profile inquiries, all of which highlighted inadequate service provision and poor co-operation for those receiving mental health care, particularly for those who had left hospital and who were thought to be a risk. At the time of the introduction of the CPA there was a separation of health and social services, and confusion, duplication of roles and a climate of risk consciousness.

Since its introduction, the CPA has undergone a number of reviews and changes, the first of which followed the case of Christopher Clunis, who stabbed to death a man at Finsbury Park Tube station in December 1992. The resulting report (DH, 1994) found one failure or missed opportunity after another.

- Following Clunis, the report (DH, 1994) recommended the introduction of a supervision register. A year later, *Building Bridges* (DH, 1995) was published and defined the four main elements of the CPA:
  - assessment
  - a care plan
  - care co-ordination
  - review.

■ In 1999, *Effective Care Co-ordination in Mental Health Services* (DH, 1999) cemented the relationship between the CPA and care management, and two levels of the CPA, standard and enhanced, were introduced with the requirement that care plans would be reviewed at least every six months and be subject to regular audit. The supervision register was abolished, which had become unpopular and was criticised as it was more likely to be applied to black and other ethnic minority groups.

■ The most recent change to the CPA occurred in 2008 with the publishing of Refocusing the Care Programme Approach (DH, 2008). This ended the two levels of the CPA and targeted only those defined as complex or high risk and whose care was being provided across agencies.

Now with just one category, for people with depression and/or anxiety, only the most severely ill and those who are considered to be at risk will be subject to the CPA. The CPA is an integral component of all mental health services, and on a practical level the CPA has four stages:

■ **Assessment.** The purpose of an assessment is designed to establish a person's needs and should receive input from the whole team. Assessment will include the person's mental and physical health, their behaviours, their risk to self and others, their support structures such as housing and employment and the person's financial circumstances such as dependants.

■ **Care plan.** The care plan brings together how people are going to respond to and manage the individual's needs. It also provides a measure of the individual's progress or deterioration. The service user should be part of the process of writing the care plan, and their wishes should be considered, both now and in the future in case they deteriorate to the point that they are no longer able to advocate for themselves.

■ **Appointing a care co-ordinator.** The care co-ordinator is the first point of contact between the service user and various health and social care professionals involved in the person's assessment and treatment.

■ **Review.** Reviews consider the assessment of the whole team. It is a dynamic process and will consider changing circumstances and the implications for the individual's care plan, and what changes are required to continue to meet that person's needs. To assist the person and consider their needs it is good practice to have support, if required, in the form of a friend, carer or advocate. Reviews should be held according to the person's needs, and at least every six months.

The following case studies illustrate how the CPA is used in practice.

Case study: Jane

Jane is a 20-year-old woman with ID. Until recently she was living in her own flat with a few hours of outreach support every other day.

Jane is now a patient on a specialist inpatient service for people with ID. She was admitted under Section 2 of the Mental Health Act (2007) for assessment. For a couple of months leading up to admission there had been a significant and gradual deterioration in Jane's functioning. She stopped attending college classes, refused to see her friends and family, her mood was consistently low and she had a reduced appetite, with consequential weight loss and disturbed sleep. She was also not managing in her flat, even with outreach support. Her home was very messy, which was unusual for Jane, and the kitchen was very unhygienic.

She was seen by the consultant psychiatrist from the local mental health in intellectual disabilities team, who also suspected that Jane was experiencing some psychotic symptoms, such as delusions of guilt, and she also reported frequent suicidal ideation. They recommended a Mental Health Act assessment as Jane did not agree with the idea of a hospital admission. After two weeks of admission, Jane was transferred onto a Section 3 for treatment of severe depression with psychotic symptoms.

CPA throughout admission

On admission, Jane was given a primary nurse, who was also her CPA care co-ordinator during her time on the ward. Jane's first CPA meeting was booked for six weeks after admission. Leading up to the meeting the primary nurse regularly met with Jane to complete the CPA assessment, which looked at many areas of life affecting mental health. With Jane's permission the primary nurse also liaised with the outreach staff, Jane's mother and her community psychiatric nurse (CPN) as part of the assessment. Clinicians from the ward were also consulted, such as the occupational therapist, consultant psychiatrist, psychologist and nursing team.

continued >

From the assessment, Jane and her primary nurse devised a care plan that:

- educated Jane about her mental health problem and her treatment
- introduced interventions to support Jane to manage her psychotic experiences
- introduced a gradual programme of activities on the ward, including cookery, social skills and exercise
- began planning for discharge and assessed the level of support Jane would need when she returned to the community.

CPA on discharge

Throughout her admission Jane had a CPA review every six weeks, which gave updates on progress and amended care plans as needed, as well as making plans for discharge. After four months of admission a discharge date was planned.

At the CPA discharge meeting it was agreed that her CPN would become Jane's CPA care co-ordinator. Care plans were agreed that would support Jane's move back into her flat, with an increased amount of outreach, a referral to community psychology services and a range of interventions to promote Jane's mental health. The CPA also made a crisis plan, identifying early signs of relapse, which was to be actioned if such a relapse was to occur. The CPA was agreed and signed by Jane, her mother and both the inpatient primary nurse and CPN.

Case study: Ben

Ben is a 52-year-old man with ID. He lives in a house that he shares with three other people with 24-hour staff support. Ben has epilepsy, which had been difficult to manage until he started a new medication. He was also being seeing a physiotherapist due to an injury he sustained after falling over.

Ben started to feel low and at the same time began to experience symptoms of anxiety including sleeplessness, loss of appetite and intrusive thoughts about hurting himself. He also experienced nausea, tremors, frequent headaches, over tiredness, insomnia and irritability. The staff team initially thought these experiences were related to his epilepsy and the frequent seizures he was experiencing. However, the symptoms have continued even though his epilepsy has been well managed.

continued >

Ben's episodes of anxiety can occur at anytime. Sometimes they are in response to times of stress and at other times they appear out of the blue. Recently, Ben has been experiencing these feelings most days of the week and his mood has deteriorated. He has been isolating himself in his bedroom, neglecting himself and not engaging in his normal activities or routine, even to fulfil his basic needs such as eating and drinking. The staff team thinks this has severely affected Ben's quality of life. The team referred him to a community learning disability team.

Ben was seen by both the consultant psychiatrist and consultant clinical psychologist. Following the assessment it was concluded that he was experiencing depression and had a generalised anxiety disorder. It was decided that he would benefit from a short admission for assessment under the Mental Health Act (2007) where he would be subject to the CPA. This was to allow a multidisciplinary approach in controlled conditions. It was decided that, as the psychology team would be working more closely with Ben post-discharge, they were best placed to co-ordinate care.

During the admission the assessment was aimed at developing a care plan that would meet Ben's needs and reduce a potential risk. His initial care package was as follows:

- commence anti-depressant treatment
- begin a course of assessment with a view to CBT sessions
- introduce a structured plan to support Ben to re-engage in his activities and routines, which would be supported by the staff team and a behaviour support specialist
- introduce relaxation exercises that the staff team could practice with Ben
- monitor and encourage activities for daily living.

After a six week admission, a CPA meeting was held and a care plan was made to look at both needs and risk, particularly the risk of relapse. The psychologist remained Ben's main contact. Ben's medication was reviewed by the psychiatrist, with the CPN following up in the home to keep an eye on any fluctuations in his mental state. CPA meetings were scheduled initially for every three months. After a year, Ben was free of symptoms of depression and was managing his anxiety with support.

Implementation of the CPA

Although well established, the evidence of the effectiveness of the CPA's implementation has been questioned (Simpson *et al*, 2003), with concerns being raised over the ability of services to provide effective case management. Although the CPA is a requirement, there are also concerns that it is not appropriate for people with ID, as less formal safeguards are in place. There are a number of good examples of the implementation of the CPA, such as Ali *et al* (2006), who developed a CPA audit cycle that was introduced within an ID service. Its objective was to evaluate the quality of the CPA and to improve its implementation. The project demonstrated the need for appropriate quality audits by showing how it had influenced progress over a four-year period and developed an up-to-date and robust CPA system in two inner London services.

Another good example of a collaborative approach with service users from the same team is described by Hall *et al* (2009), who reported a project put in place to ensure that issues that posed a problem for service users were identified and acted upon to make the CPA process more personal and accessible. Some of the issues identified were:

- there were too many people at the CPA meetings
- there was a lack of understanding of what was being said
- the length of the meetings
- general satisfaction with the meetings.

Following this, the group suggested solutions to make meetings more accessible. These included giving a choice of where they should be held, using easy-read care plans, imposing a limit on the number of people at the meetings, making sure that the meetings are taken more slowly, and improving the punctuality of meetings.

For people with ID, the CPA is monitored as part of the Green Light Toolkit (GLTK) (FPLD, 2004), which sets the standards for access to and the provision of mental health services for people with ID against which mental health services, social care providers and commissioners are measured.

This now forms part of the star ratings for trusts, which are required to rate themselves using a traffic light system: red meaning not achieved, amber partially achieved and green achieved. The National Services Framework was followed by *New Horizons* (DH, 2009), which introduced the recovery model. This has since been replaced by *No Health without Mental Health* (DH, 2011), which aims to reduce stigma by getting people to consider mental health in the same way as they do physical health.

Conclusion

Although it is difficult to define case management and compare the effectiveness of different models, it appears that multi-agency approaches in general are more effective. The original models have been transformed into a number of different approaches that we define as case management because of the common characteristics they share. There is, however, little evidence of the use and effectiveness of case management for people with ID. The CPA has formalised the case management approach and it is the right of everyone to be afforded the safeguards it offers. It is applied to those with mental illness regardless of diagnosis who are considered a risk to themselves or others. In terms of depression and anxiety, it is only the most complex and enduring presentations that are subject to the CPA, where they are considered at risk or a risk.

Summary

- Case management comes from the early philosophy-driven community models of the US. While we have seen both generic and more intensive teams develop in the UK, the function of these teams is often blurred and they have in some areas become indistinguishable in terms of service delivery. This has caused problems for research and the ability to identify preferred models of community care.

- The CPA came about because of a lack of joined-up care both locally and across the country, causing people who were or had been considered a danger to themselves or others to fall between gaps, at times with grave consequences. The CPA formalised case management and offered a framework for agencies to work together to plan care relating to the person's mental health and their risk to self or others.

- The CPA applies to all people. This is regardless of what additional support or frameworks may be present.

References

Agranoff R (1977) Services integration. In: W Anderson, B Frieden and M Murphy (Eds) *Managing Human Services*. Washington, DC: International City Management Association.

Ali A, Hall I, Taylor C, Attard S & Hassiotis A (2006) Auditing the care programme approach for people with learning disability: a four year audit cycle. *Psychiatric Bulletin* **30** (11) 415–418.

Burns T, Creed F, Fahy T, Thompson S, Tyrer P & White I (1999) Intensive versus standard case management for severe psychotic illness: a randomised trial. *Lancet* **353** (9171) 2185–2189.

Department of Health (1994) LASSL (94)4: Guidance on the Discharge of Mentally Disordered People and their Continuing Care in the Community [online] Department of Health. Available at: http://www.dh.gov.uk/en/Publicationsandstatistics/Lettersandcirculars/Localauthoritysocialservicesletters/AllLASSLs/DH_4003977 (accessed March 2012).

Department of Health (1995) *Building Bridges*. London: Department of Health.

Department of Health (1999) *Effective Care Co-ordination in Mental Health Services: Modernising the care programme approach*. London: Department of Health.

Department of Health (2008) *Refocusing the Care Programme Approach*. London: Department of Health.

Department of Health (2009) *New Horizons: A shared vision for mental health*. London: Department of Health.

Department of Health (2011) *No Health without Mental Health*. London: Department of Health.

FPLD (2004) *Green Light For Mental Health: How good are your mental health services for people with learning disabilities? A service improvement toolkit*. London: Foundation for People with Learning Disabilities.

Gensichen J, Torge M, Peitz M, Wendt-Hermainski H, Beyer M, Rosemann T, Krauth C, Raspe H, Aldenhoff J & Gerlach F (2005) *Case management for the treatment of patients with major depression in general practices – rationale, design and conduct of a cluster randomised controlled trial – PRoMPT (PRimary care Monitoring for depressive Patient's Trial) [ISRCTN66386086] – study protocol* [online]. BMC Public Health. Available at: http://www.biomedcentral.com/1471-2458/5/101 (accessed March 2012).

Gensichen J, von Korff M, Peitz M, Muth C, Beyer M, Güthlin C, Torge M, Petersen J, Rosemann T, König J & Gerlach F (2009) Case management for depression by health care assistants in small primary care practices: a cluster randomised trial. *Annals of International Medicine* **151** (6) 369–378.

Hall I, Burns E, Martin S, Carter E, Macreath S, Pearson M & Hassiotis A (2009) Making care programme approach meetings more accessible and person-centred for people with learning disabilities. *Advances in Mental Health and Intellectual Disabilities* **3** (1) 23–29.

Hassiotis A, Ukoumunne O, Tyrer P, Piachaud J, Harvey K, Gilvarry C, Harvey K & Fraser J (1999) Prevalence and characteristics of patients with severe mental illness and borderline intellectual functioning: report from the UK 700 randomised controlled trial of case management. *British Journal of Psychiatry* **175** 135–140.

Hassiotis A, Ukoumunne O, Byford S, Tyrer P, Harvey K, Piachaud J, Gilvarry C & Fraser J (2001) Intellectual functioning and outcome of patients with severe psychotic illness randomised to intensive case management: report from the UK 700 case management trial. *British Journal of Psychiatry* **178** 166–71.

Intagliata J (1982) Improving the quality of community care for the chronically mentally disabled: the role of case management. *Schizophrenia Bulletin* **8** (4) 655–674.

Marshall M, Gray A, Lockwood A & Green R (1998) Case management for people with severe mental disorders. *The Cochrane Database of Systematic Reviews* (4) CD000050.

Muijen M, Marks I, Connolly J, Audini B & McNamee G (1992) The Daily Living Programme. Preliminary comparison of community versus hospital-based treatment for the seriously mentally ill facing emergency admission. *British Journal of Psychiatry* **160** 379–384.

Muijen M, Cooney M, Strathdee G, Bell R & Hudson A (1994) Community psychiatric nurse teams: intensive support versus generic care. *British Journal of Psychiatry* **165** 211–217.

Moore S (1960) A psychiatric outpatient nursing service. *Mental Health Bulletin* **20** 51–54.

Moore S (1964) Mental nursing in the community. *Nursing Times* **60** 467–470.

Simpson A, Miller C & Bowers L (2003) The history of the care programme approach in England: where did it go wrong? *Journal of mental health* **12** (5) 489–504.

Smith L & Newton R (2007) Systematic review of case management. *Australian and New Zealand Journal of Psychiatry* **41** (4) 2–9.

Stein L & Test M (1980) Alternatives to mental hospital treatment. I. Conceptual model, treatment programme and clinical evaluation. *Archives of General Psychiatry* **37** (4) 392–397.

Thompson K, Griffith E & Leaf P (1990) A historical review of the Madison model of community care. *Hospital and Community Psychiatry* **41** (6) 625–634.

Williams J Jr, Gerrity M, Holsinger T, Dobscha S, Gaynes B & Dietrich A (2007) Systematic review of multifaceted interventions to improve depression care. *General Hospital Psychiatry* **29** (2) 91–116.

Chapter 12

Intensive support teams

Sue Freeman and Philip Reynolds

Overview

People with ID experiencing anxiety and/or depression should be offered the same options for intervention as the rest of the population, however in reality this is often not the case. The current vision, whereby people should have access to mainstream services, can often prove difficult to achieve and for some people there is a need for support from specialist ID services. This is most effective when it is provided in the form of intense support. This chapter examines how intense specialist support, provided by a team of multidisciplinary professionals, can achieve positive outcomes for people with ID experiencing anxiety and/or depression by offering a wide range of adapted therapies. It describes how the team can work together flexibly across multiple environments, including with mainstream services in partnership with the individual and their carers.

Learning objectives

- To be aware of how intensive support services that focus on supporting people with ID and challenging behaviour are essential to modern learning disability services.

- Understand the importance of multidisciplinary formulation and intervention when supporting people with anxiety and/or depression.

- Identify the importance of a continuous care pathway between inpatient and community services.

Introduction

The white paper *Valuing People* (DH, 2001) set out the government's vision for people with ID and includes their health needs as a central part of this vision. It states that all people with ID will have equal access to mainstream health services, and identifies that in order to address the mental health needs of people with ID, mainstream mental health services will need to become more responsive while specialist ID services will need to provide facilitation and support. However, the white paper acknowledged the need for specialist ID inpatient services for a small number of people who are unable to access mainstream services, even with support and reasonable adjustment.

In reality, mainstream mental health services often struggle to support people with ID, which leads to the overshadowing of the extent of their mental health problems. Where mental health needs are identified, people with ID are often restricted from being offered the full range of support that is offered to the rest of the population.

The *National Service Framework for Mental Health* (DH, 1999) set out clear and nationally agreed care standards expected from mental health services, and it applied to all adults of working age. A self-assessment (autumn assessment) enabled local mental health implementation teams to monitor progress against this framework, and includes assessing the availability of assertive outreach, acute inpatient services and the use of the Care Programme Approach (CPA). The assessment covered 41 aspects of service provision. Number 40, added in 2003, aimed to monitor the application of the National Service Framework to people with ID who have mental health problems. The Green Light Toolkit (GLTK) was developed in 2004 in support of the implementation of this standard and aimed to address the inequalities for people with ID (FDLP, 2004). The GLTK is a self-assessment tool designed to be used between different partnerships including commissioners, carers, people with ID and providers.Traditionally, community support has been provided for people with ID by specialist learning disability teams. This involves supporting people with mental health needs, including helping them to access mainstream services. However, community teams provide for the whole range of generic learning disability services, and mental health and challenging behaviour are only a small part of their work. This area is not, therefore, seen as the main priority. Often there are tensions between team members, some believing that mental health and challenging behaviour stigmatises the majority of clients and takes up too many of the team's resources (Hassiotis *et al*, 2003). This results in a stagnation in the growth of intervention and a shortage of skilled professionals to work with this client group, particularly in community settings (Hassiotis *et al*, 2003).

Community teams often support people with challenging behaviour and/or mental health needs (Slevin *et al*, 2008), however there is a need for further intensive support and skill sets across all community settings. This belief is reinforced by Mansell (DH, 2007), who states that additional specialist multidisciplinary teams focused on mental health and/or challenging behaviour are an essential component of modern provision, recognising that the intensity and complexity of help required may be more than that which the community learning disability teams can provide.

One approach to providing intense support has been to develop assertive specialist learning disability community teams, which work in partnership with and complement mental health services and community teams, delivering intensive and assertive outreach support to people with ID and mental health needs with or without challenging behaviour.

Assertive community treatment (ACT) was developed in the early 1970s as a means of co-ordinating the care of people with severe mental illness in the community. A Cochrane review of the effectiveness of ACT for the general population found that people receiving ACT were less like to be admitted into inpatient care and more likely to engage with services (Prakash *et al*, 2007). The National Service Framework (DH, 1999) and the NHS Plan (DH, 2000) called for a total of 220 assertive outreach teams. This approach has been adopted within learning disability services and has been further developed to include intense support to people whose behaviour challenges services. However, the model of intensive support varies across the UK.

Intensive support service

The Intensive Support Service (ISS) in Northamptonshire provides specialist support to people with ID who challenge services, with or without mental health needs, using four local community teams. The service model was developed in 2009 in response to a number of pieces of national policy, including *Valuing People* (DH, 2001), the Mansell Report (DH, 2007) and *New Horizons* (DH, 2009). It provides intensive specialist assessment, formulation, intervention and direct training to care staff over and above that which can be offered by local community teams. The ISS is set up to respond to people whose needs require intensive case management, support and engagement, and it works in partnership with the community team for people with learning disability, mental health services, local authorities and other mainstream services in an attempt to provide a seamless service.

The ISS consists of a four-bedded inpatient assessment and treatment unit (ATU) and an outreach Intensive Support Team (IST). The service is multidisciplinary and includes a psychiatrist, psychologist and senior assistant psychologist, speech and language therapist, occupational therapist, nurse behaviour therapist, nurse consultant, nurses and healthcare assistants. The team is managed jointly by the nurse consultant and principal clinical psychologist, which provides strong clinical leadership that is committed to the social model of disability and the approach described in the Mansell report (DH, 2007). Knowledgeable, innovative and experienced clinical leaders who can take informed risks are crucial to successfully supporting people who challenge services (National Development Team for Inclusion, 2010).

While all people accessing the service will have a care co-ordinator (the majority being supported by the CPA (see Chapter 11)), there is a whole-team approach to care and each profession brings a different perspective to the decision-making process. The senior representation among the differing professions supports high-level decision-making, including situations where no precedent is set. This is important as it enables positive risk-taking for people with complex needs. The service is principally community based, aiming to address people's presenting difficulties while maintaining meaningful links with their social and material environments, as well as their friends and family.

It is recognised that there are occasions when the level of risk prevents a person from continuing to be supported in the community and needs a short-term inpatient admission. Individuals who are not able to be supported in mainstream services with reasonable adjustments are admitted to the ISS's ATU, which strives to continue to provide as close to normal living conditions as possible and has on site a therapy room, training kitchen, gym, gardens and canteen.

The integrated working between the ATU and the IST enables both in-reach and outreach intervention across specialist and mainstream services. The team also provides assertive outreach to those people who are hard to engage. This level of support leads to the successful outcomes achieved by the service. This type of support has been identified as successfully reducing the length of inpatient stay for people with mental health needs and low IQ (Hassiotis *et al*, 2001). As identified by Slevin *et al* (2008), the success of inpatient admissions depends on effective community based support when the person is discharged.

The seamless process offered by the ISS enables positive outcomes to be achieved, as has been demonstrated by the use of the Health of the Nation Outcome Scales for People with Learning Disabilities (HoNOS–LD), which is an outcome tool developed for people with ID whereby the person is rated by the clinician with information from someone who knows the client well. The behaviours identified are rated over a four-week period and these ratings can then be monitored over time to identify changes in behaviour and mental health.

Using HoNOS–LD, initial scores show an overall decrease of 88% in symptoms reported on referral for the total number of patients who access the service. This is an average individual decrease of 6.5 points, which represents a clinically significant decrease. Referrals to the ISS are usually complex in nature and can be further complicated by the fact that mental health issues may coexist with challenging behaviour, whether it is an expression of mental illness or not (Taggart & Slevin, 2006).

Another common co-morbid condition is autism. It is estimated that 20–33% of adults with ID have autism (Emerson & Baines, 2010), and a significant number of people referred to the ISS are identified as having an autism spectrum disorder. A study by Bradley and Bolton (2006) in relation to teenagers with autism found that teenagers with both ID and autism were likely to have higher rates of episodic psychiatric disorders than those with ID alone. Bakken *et al* (2010), meanwhile, found that people with autism are more likely to have anxiety related conditions, and Gillott (2004) suggests that people with autism are almost three times more anxious than their non-autistic peers.

As a secondary specialist service, the ISS sets out to deliver health interventions to individuals with varyingly complex needs, and works within the recovery approach. In addition, the team often supports a person to improve their adaptive functioning and supports changes in the home and community environment. It has a detailed and flexible care pathway that aims to meet the needs of the client group offering evidence-based interventions.

Working as a multidisciplinary team

The following case examples will endeavour to demonstrate both the work of the ISS's inpatient unit and its community based team, and indeed the close collaboration of the two. Combining these two elements works on the assumption that, for those people whose behaviour has challenged services or the environments in which they live, any one approach in isolation would be unlikely to succeed. Interventions, therefore, will need to draw on the expertise, skills and experience of a number of professions in a co-ordinated and unified fashion.

Central to the first element, is the use of a shared formulation. Kennedy (2009) highlights the need for formulation in inpatient settings, saying: '*a successful inpatient intervention needs to teach new behaviours, thoughts, feelings and physiological responses in the inpatient context and then enable transfer of these new skills to the natural environment in which the client normally exists … formulation is necessary for both environments, enabling predictions as to what might change when the environments, with their differing contingencies, change*' (p44). We would also argue that the value of formulation applies to community intervention, because the skills taught during intervention need to translate to the environment and be maintained when the professionals are no longer involved. So again, predications need to be made on the basis of formulations as to the likely outcomes at the end of a period of intervention. It is important that the professionals involved share this formulation so that they are working to the same ends with the same goals in mind.

Case study: James

James, a 22-year-old man, was referred to the ISS by a consultant psychiatrist from a local community team for people with learning disability. He was presenting with high levels of aggression directed at his family, problems with excessive alcohol consumption, possible trauma and possible psychosis.

James has mild ID. He attended an special educational needs (SEN) school until he was 18, and while he reported that he enjoyed his time there he did not sit any exams. Since school he has had no permanent work, education or day placement, and had spent most of his time at home. It seemed that he had a college placement arranged but he chose not to take this up. His mother reported a history of aggressive behaviour from childhood but that this has been significantly worse in recent times. She also reported two particularly distressing experiences for James, one when he was attacked by a group of people in the local park and one where he was subject to a serious assault from an older man.

James, however, gave very little detail about either incident and found it difficult to talk about them at assessment. This information was initially provided by the family. However, during the course of treatment he was able to say that it was his thoughts about these events that caused him to be anxious.

He had been diagnosed with schizoaffective disorder in the past, but this was questioned by the psychiatrist at the time of his referral to the ISS.

Assessment

Following an out-patient appointment, James was admitted to the ATU for a mental health assessment. He was in hospital for four weeks and during this time there was no evidence of schizoaffective disorder and no clinical management problems were observed. At this point the IST became involved, with the case holder spending time on the ATU building up a therapeutic relationship and explaining their role in preparation for when James returned to his home environment. The assessment during his admission included monitoring his mental state by the psychiatrist, who ruled out schizoaffective disorder.

continued >

From the initial assessment on the ATU it was clear that he was in fact relatively settled during the admission and enjoyed his time on the ward. He started to express that he felt comfortable and safe away from his home environment, and without access to alcohol there was no evidence of aggression during the admission. James was initially reluctant to talk to the clinical psychologist involved, but as he started to discuss his difficulties he described significant levels of anxiety, with panic attacks at times when in the community. These experiences of anxiety were also observed by ISS staff when out with James. On discussion, it seemed that James' thoughts during these panic attacks were related to the distressing events that his mum had mentioned but which he found difficult to talk about. He was only willing to indicate that his distress was linked to these thoughts but was not willing to talk about them in more detail. Although it was clear that he struggled to develop relationships with males, he did develop a therapeutic relationship with both the male clinical psychologist and a male nurse from the team with support from the female nurse behaviour therapist.

Formulation

The working formulation was that James was a young man with a mild learning disability and 48 XXYY genetic syndrome who had a complex family background and a history of aggressive behaviour, but that his drinking problem and aggression were precipitated by a combination of traumatic events that have left him with significant anxieties and PTSD. McCarthy (2001) quoted aggression as one of the most common symptoms exhibited by people with ID as a consequence of PTSD. PTSD was formulated using Ehlers and Clark's (2000) cognitive model of PTSD in which the danger from past events is experienced as a present threat due to cognitive biases that act to increase the perceived threat.

He was also believed to be using alcohol to manage his anxieties and this exacerbated his aggression, however the relief from his anxieties provided by the alcohol maintained the problem. His family situation also acted to maintain his anxiety as it could be chaotic at times and was unable to contain his anxiety. Other family members would at times be living in the house and many family members and friends could be in and out of the house. This, along with other stressful events within the family, added to the unpredictability of his life.

continued >

Intervention

A team consisting of a clinical psychologist, nurse behaviour therapist, a specialist learning disability nurse and a support worker worked with James over a 12-month period. The intervention was structured around CBT, adapted for people with ID using an approach discussed by Lindsay (1999) and Kroese (1998).

The family had no previous contact with services, and therefore the initial task was to develop a therapeutic relationship with them, explaining roles, responsibilities and services available. James was supported to develop a person centred plan (PCP) and this was an avenue to further develop a therapeutic relationship with him. James worked on his PCP with the nurse behaviour therapist, and this process involved him being supported to consider what his goals were for the future, how he could start to work towards them and the type of support he needed both professionally and in terms of family and friends. James met weekly with the ISS psychologist, who was male, supported by the female case holder.

The intervention plan had initially been to work with James to develop coping skills, and then to work directly with the past traumatic experiences. James was, however, unwilling or unable at that point in time to discuss the content of his thoughts in detail, but he was able to express that the content was linked to his previous traumatic experiences. Although he was not willing to look in detail at his past experiences, he was willing to be supported with his anxieties and to look in general at the impacts of trauma.

The model of PTSD was discussed with him and he gained an understanding of how his past experiences had impacted on his current anxieties. The PTSD model was discussed using the analogy of memory as a cupboard in which your memories are stored on the shelves. Bad or traumatic memories are not neatly placed on the shelves but rather stuffed into the cupboard and the doors slammed shut leaving the doors to fall open at unpredictable times and those bad memories to fall out only to be stuffed back in again and never looked at in detail or placed on a shelf with the rest of your memories. This analogy was supported with visual representations and a demonstration with a cupboard to reduce the abstract nature of the model. James was aware that if he did want to discuss his past he was able to do this at any point, and we worked on coping skills to deal with difficult emotions as they came up.

continued >

As James was unwilling to talk directly about his traumatic experiences, the intervention plan was revised and a CBT approach was used, as mentioned, to look at the anxiety symptoms rather than to work directly with the past traumatic memories. James was supported to discuss the situations in which he was anxious and to develop a visual rating scale so that he could start to consider which situations were more difficult than others. He identified going into town, into parks or into certain shops as the main situations he feared. In general he was fearful of many situations where there may have been groups of people about.

Once James was able to start thinking about these situations, the team was able to help him to develop a graded hierarchy of anxiety-provoking situations, which he would be supported to expose himself to while his anxiety before, during and following the exposure sessions was monitored. His experience and ratings were then used as a discussion point in sessions to help him understand his anxieties, challenge his thoughts, develop confidence and discuss future goals for his graded exposure. These exposure sessions were initially on a twice-weekly basis with an additional weekly session to discuss these experiences.

James' engagement was not always consistent, and at times the team had to cancel and rearrange sessions when he was not willing to engage. The team had to negotiate therapeutic goals and support the family to encourage James, but only at his own pace. The team also supported the family by meeting with them, with James' consent, and explaining to them that James needed to be encouraged to work on his graded exposure but that it needed to be under his control. The family was also practically supported in order to attend meetings that helped James, and they were given information about local services for financial support. This gradual approach gained James' trust and he was able to work up his graded hierarchy, gaining in confidence and reducing his anxiety.

James attended CAN, a local substance misuse service, usually with the support of an IST nurse, however he did attend some of the sessions independently. James' alcohol dependency and intake declined as his anxiety reduced, as did his level of aggression. This was monitored by self-report from James and also confirmed by the family's report.

continued >

While the focus of the work was on graded exposure, the team also worked to support him looking at his accommodation. He looked into the option of living on his own with support, however he chose to remain at home. He also explored opportunities outside of the home and attended a horticultural course with support for a number of weeks. James also became keen to look at his physical health, and so he was supported to engage with a nurse in the community team, which proved successful when previously he had refused to engage with services.

Outcome

There was a significant decrease in James' alcohol consumption and a decrease in his aggression within the family home. He gained skills to reflect, recognise and monitor his anxiety, and he developed the ability to solve problems and set his own goals. James appeared more confident and improved his communication skills. He appeared to be making clear choices and expressed enjoying being in control of his life.

Using HoNOS–LD, which is used regularly by the ISS to monitor outcomes, James' scores reduced from 27 to eight during the period of intervention, demonstrating a clinically significant change in his presentation and a positive outcome for James.

Case study: Mark

Mark was a 23-year-old man who was referred to the ISS via a call to the duty clinician because he was in crisis. He was very distressed and was behaving aggressively towards his parents. He had caused damage at home and had hidden objects in his room that could have been used as weapons. Initially no bed was available on the learning disability ATU, and so Mark was admitted for one day to his local mental health ATU with liaison from the ISS and then transferred when a bed became available.

Mark had a mild ID and autism. He attended an SEN school until he was 16, when he transferred to a mainstream local sixth form college.

continued >

Assessment

Mark was admitted to the ATU for assessment of his challenging behaviour and mental health. It was apparent that Mark was extremely anxious and initially withdrew from the open ward environment to his bedroom. People with autism can exhibit higher levels of social anxiety than other non-autistic peers, most likely due to fear and worry regarding social situations (Gobrial & Raghavan, unpublished). At home it was reported that he had become increasingly mistrusting of other people. When he did feel comfortable enough to discuss his worries he also discussed a great sense of shame at his behaviour towards his parents and a feeling of hopelessness about his ability to move forward with his life. He was presenting with both high levels of anxiety and depression.

As he opened up more to staff and started to discuss his fears he was also able to start discussing his perception that people were staring at him or laughing at him. This perception could apply to strangers who he saw while out but also to co-patients on the ward and members of staff who were working with him. It also became clear that he found it difficult to understand and recognise emotions, making it more likely that he may make a negative assumption about people's emotions such as them being angry or aggressive.

His parents reported that he had enjoyed his time at the SEN school but had struggled at a mainstream college. His parents also reported that his behaviour had started to change while he was at college, and he reported being bullied. These experiences seemed to have had an impact on his confidence and on his ability to trust people. His placement at college had broken down due to the bullying, and he then had numerous support workers and changes to his care package.

During the year leading up to the admission, Mark's anxiety levels had appeared to increase and this had also led to an increase in ritualistic behaviour. He had also started to believe that people in the community were laughing at him, and he started to throw objects about at home and be both verbally and physically aggressive towards his parents.

Formulation

The working formulation that was developed was that Mark was a young man with a mild ID and autism who had experienced a very difficult transition from an SEN school to a mainstream college.

continued >

Here, the general environment, lack of structure compared to his previous school, and in particular his experience of bullying, created a great deal of stress for Mark, which developed into anxiety, specifically presenting as a social phobia. As stated, the co-existence of depression, agoraphobia and social phobia are common in people with PTSD (Brady, 1997) and autism.

Collishaw *et al* (2004) have identified that challenging behaviour in people with ID is often associated with the experience of critical life events. The impact of the social phobia and the perception that people were laughing or staring at him also had a significant impact on his mood, leading to depression. His reflections on his behaviour also lead him to feel ashamed, which increased his depressed mood, as is common among people with PTSD (Andrews, 1998). His difficulty with understanding and recognising emotions was also hypothesised to play a significant role in maintaining his difficulties and contributed to a developing sense that people were against him. He also had limited skills to cope with difficult emotions, which again contributed to the development of challenging behaviour as a coping mechanism that kept the threats he perceived in the world at bay.

Intervention

The multidisciplinary team that worked with Mark on the ATU included the nursing team, a clinical psychologist, an assistant clinical psychologist, a psychiatrist, an occupational therapist and a speech and language therapist. The approach that was used drew on an adapted CBT approach, but in this case significant attention needed to be paid to the barriers to using CBT identified by Kroese (1998), such as a poor ability to self-report, a lack of understanding of abstract concepts and the environment's lack of ability to support self-regulation.

The intervention focused on a number of areas following on from the formulation. These included helping Mark to understand emotions and to apply this understanding to other people's emotions, and encouraging him to express his own emotions, thus tackling the first barrier to CBT identified above – the ability to self-report. The 'Mind Reading Program' developed by Simon Baron-Cohen (2007) is a DVD-based resource that uses video and audio clips in a game-based format to teach the basics of emotions.

continued >

This program was used by a nurse from the IST while Mark was still an inpatient, and when discharged it was used as a starting point to help teach Mark about emotions. He engaged well using this approach. Examples from magazines and TV programmes were then used to help Mark generalise what he had learnt about emotions.

Desensitisation and exposure therapy are effective management strategies in social phobia. Some studies suggest that optimum results are achieved by combining psychological and pharmacological interventions (Cooray & Bakala, 2005). The team therefore also worked to engage Mark in activities to help him challenge his assumptions and develop his independence, confidence and self-esteem while providing graded exposure to those social situations that he was fearful of. This also addressed the second barrier to CBT by making abstract concepts concrete by basing discussions on real experience.

The psychiatrist, meanwhile, regularly monitored his mood, both in hospital and on discharge, and prescribed medication using a low dose of risperidone (0.25mg) to help reduce his anxiety in the short term and thus provide a window of opportunity to develop the therapeutic intervention. The speech and language therapist worked with Mark and his family, and the nursing team, in order to develop social stories to help him understand his current situation and then to help with key transitions, such as extending his time outside of the unit and working towards being discharged home.

The nursing team on the unit worked to help Mark structure his day and engage in graded activities. One health care assistant in particular developed a good rapport with Mark and gained his trust, enabling him to encourage Mark to work with the rest of the team. The activities the nursing team helped him engage in exposed him to his fear of social situations, building up from spending time in shared ward spaces to using the hospital grounds and canteen, and ultimately to spending time in the community and local shops.

The assistant clinical psychologist discussed Mark's worries with him in order to gain a better understanding of his fears from his perspective and where they had come from. In this way the assistant clinical psychologist was able to help Mark work towards challenging his thoughts and fears by drawing on his new experiences from the graded exposure work.

continued >

The clinical psychologist worked closely with the team to develop the graded exposure programme and advised on the work that helped Mark to better understand emotions. He also worked with the family to discuss their worries and help them understand the formulation of the problem and express their previous and current emotions. A nurse from the intensive support team also started to work with Mark during his admission, to aid a smooth discharge and continue treatment into the community.

Mark's family was also heavily involved in the intervention and this helped to address the final barrier to using CBT – the environment's ability to support self-regulation. The family initially needed to express their concerns and share their experiences with professionals. Since discharge, the family has stressed how it would have been helpful to talk to other families that had been through similar experiences, as at the time they felt alone in their experience. The parents worked with the team to develop an activity schedule and social stories to support reintegration activities. Work was also done with the family to increase his independence. Both Mark and his parents were closely involved in discussing the next steps in his exposure programme and in monitoring his progress.

The team worked with Mark to build up relationships with the staff who would be supporting him on discharge so that he felt comfortable with them and so that they were involved in the graded exposure from an early stage. The staff that would be supporting him started to visit him and work with him while he was in the unit to develop a relationship with him, and they started to become involved with his treatment, meeting with the family and supporting home visits.

Occupational therapy sessions also started while Mark was in hospital, looking at activities that he enjoyed and also developing skills, such as baking, which he particularly enjoyed. These sessions were an important contribution to improving his mood by giving him the opportunity to engage in activities for pleasure and to develop skills that gave him a sense of mastery. These sessions also continued at home with the occupational therapist, who was able to follow Mark through from the inpatient unit to home.

continued >

Towards discharge, a well-being plan was developed with Mark, who identified the things in his life that helped to keep him well, signs that things were deteriorating and those things he could do if he was finding things difficult again in the future.

Outcome

At the end of the interventions Mark was more confident, able to recognise his emotions, manage his anxieties and talk about his worries and fears when he needed to. He was happy to use his well-being plan. Mark had re-established a full timetable of activities that included walking, rock climbing, sailing and cooking, as well as accessing regular respite care.

Again, using the HoNOS–LD, Mark's progress was captured with scores reducing from 32 to three during the period of intervention.

Conclusion

People with ID can be offered a wide range of interventions, with some adaptations, for anxiety and depression. It is important that interventions focus on biological, psychological and social factors. Due to the intensive nature of interventions, the provision of specialist learning disability intensive support is essential, as is multidisciplinary and agency working. Where the risk is high and an inpatient admission is required, it is essential that the community team provides in-reach to ensure a successful discharge. The two case studies above demonstrate the effectiveness of team working across inpatient and community settings, however more research is required in this area.

Summary

- Teams such as the IST are essential components of modern services. They provide intensive support and focus when supporting people with ID and mental health needs, thus enabling community services to continue to serve a wider diversity of need.

- It is important that the teams are multidisciplinary in nature so that assessment, formulation and intervention take into consideration biological, psychological and social factors.

■ Where people in crisis require an inpatient admission it is essential that there is a seamless care pathway between inpatient and community care in order to maximise outcomes.

References

Andrews B (1998) Shame and childhood abuse. In: P Gilbert and B Andrews (Eds) *Shame: Interpersonal behaviour, psychopathology and culture* (pp176–190). Oxford: Oxford University Press.

Bakken T, Helverschou S, Eilertsen D, Heggelund T, Myrbakk E & Martinsen H (2010) Psychiatric disorders in adolescents and adults with autism and intellectual disability: a representative study in one county in Norway. *Research in Developmental Disabilities* **31** (6) 1669–1677.

Baron-Cohen S (2007) Mind Reading: *The interactive guide to emotions*. London: Jessica Kingsley Publishers.

Brady K (1997) Post traumatic stress disorder and comorbidity: recognising the many faces of PTSD. *Journal of Clinical Psychiatry* **58** (9) 12–15.

Bradley E & Bolton P (2006) Episodic psychiatric disorders in teenagers with learning disabilities with or without autism. *British Journal of Psychiatry* **189** 361–366.

Collishaw S, Maughan B & Pickles A (2004) Affective problems in adults with mild learning disability: the roles of social disadvantage and ill health. *British Journal of Psychiatry* **185** 350–351.

Cooray S & Bakala A (2005) Anxiety disorders in people with learning disabilities. *Advances in Psychiatric Treatment* **11** 355–361.

Department of Health (1999) *National Service Framework for Mental Health: Modern standards and service models*. London: TSO.

Department of Health (2000) *The NHS Plan: A plan for investment, a plan for reform*. London: TSO.

Department of Health (2001) *Valuing People: A new strategy for learning disability for the 21st century*. London: TSO.

Department of Health (2007) *Services for People with Learning Disabilities and Challenging Behaviour or Mental Health Needs: Report of a project group* (Mansell Report) London: TSO.

Department of Health (2009) *New Horizons: A shared vision for mental health*. London: TSO.

Ehlers A & Clark D (2000) A cognitive model of posttraumatic stress disorder. *Behaviour Research and Therapy* **38** (4) 319–345.

Emerson E & Baines S (2010) *The Estimated Prevalence of Autism among Adults with Learning Disabilities in England*. Improving Health and Lives: Learning Disability Observatory. Available at: http://www.improvinghealthandlives.org.uk/uploads/doc/vid_8731_IHAL2010-05Autism.pdf (accessed March 2012).

Foundation for People with Learning Disabilities (2004) *Green Light for Mental Health: How good are your mental health services for people with learning disabilities? A service improvement toolkit*. London: Foundation for People with Learning Disabilities.

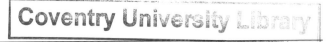

Gillott A (2004) Anxiety and stress in adults with autism. *Journal of Intellectual Disability Research* **48** 321–339.

Gobrial E & Raghavan R (2007) *Anxiety Disorders in Children with Learning Disabilities and Autism: A review* (unpublished).

Hassiotis A, Ukoumunne O, Byford S, Tyrer P, Harvey K, Piachaud J, Gilvarry K & Fraser J (2001) Intellectual functioning and outcome of patients with severe psychotic illness randomised to intensive case management: report from the UK700 trial. *British Journal of Psychiatry* **178** 166–171.

Hassiotis A, Tyrer P & Oliver P (2003) Psychiatric assertive outreach and learning disability services. *Advances in Psychiatric Treatment* **9** 368–373.

Kennedy F (2009) The use of formulation in inpatient settings. In: I Clarke and H Wilson (Eds) *Cognitive Behaviour Therapy for Acute Inpatient Mental Health Units*. London: Routledge.

Kroese B (1998) Cognitive behavioural therapy for people with learning disabilities. *Behavioural and Cognitive Psychotherapy* **26** (4) 315–322.

Lindsay W (1999) Cognitive therapy in learning disabilities and mental health. *The Psychologist* **12** (5) 238–241.

McCarthy J (2001) Post-traumatic stress disorder in people with learning disability. *Advances in Psychiatric Treatment* **7** 163–169.

National Development Team for Inclusion (2010) *Guide for Commissioners of Services for People with Learning Disabilities who Challenge Services*. Bath: NDTi.

Prakash J, Andrews T & Porter I (2007) Service innovation: assertive outreach teams for adults with learning disabilities. *The Psychiatrist Bulletin* **31** 138–141.

Slevin E, McConkey R, Truesdale-Kennedy M & Taggart L (2008) People with learning disabilities admitted to an assessment and treatment unit: impact on challenging behaviours and mental health problems. *Journal of Psychiatric and Mental Health Nursing* **15** (7) 537–546.

Taggart L & Slevin E (2006) Care planning in mental health settings. In: B Gates (Ed) *Care Planning and Delivery in Intellectual Disability Nursing* (pp158–194). Oxford: Blackwell.

Subject index

Agoraphobia 24, 25, 233

Anxiety

       Assessment 39

       Assessment instruments 39–43

       Epidemiology 31–32

       Diagnosis 35–39

       Management 117–120

Autism 119, 153, 191–201

Biological factors 34, 59

Behavioural phenotypes 30, 66

Calm Child Programme (CCP) 194–203

Care management 212

Care programme approach (CPA) 207, 211, 212

Case formulation 89

Case formulation workshops 92-99

Challenging behaviour 36, 54, 91–92, 142, 221–223, 225, 232–233

Cognitive behaviour therapy (CBT) 89–90, 92, 96, 98, 160, 229–235

Cognitive therapy 125–137

Depression

       Clinical features 53–56

       Epidemiology 57–58

       Aetiology 59–62

       Diagnostic aspects 62–66

       Assessment tools 67–69

       Management 107–117

Disablism 15

Electroconvulsive therapy (ECT) 116

Emotional problems 7, 192

Fragile X syndrome 30, 59, 70

Generalised anxiety disorder 23, 33, 118, 215

Intensive support team 221

Intensive support service 223

Light therapy 117

Mental health disorders 8–9, 16,

Mental health strategy 12

Obsessive compulsive disorder 27–30, 32–34, 39

Panic disorder 23, 25, 31, 33, 45

Pervasive developmental disorder 33, 39

Phobia 24–26, 233–234

Psychological therapies 13, 116, 135, 151

Psychodynamic perspective 159–187

Psychopharmacological approaches 105–121

Post-traumatic stress disorder 28–29, 34, 228–229, 233

Resilience 7, 15–16

Self-injurious behaviour 56–57, 64, 119

Self assessment and intervention (SAINT) 80–86

Social phobia 25

Solution focussed brief therapy 141–156

Supporting families 191

Specific phobia 26

Therapeutic relationship 13, 128, 163, 167, 169, 172, 174, 184, 227–229

User perspectives 75–87

Anxiety and Depression in People with Intellectual Disabilities © Pavilion Publishing and Media Ltd 2012